STO

DID Y

- Son
  dam

- As
  rary hearing loss owing to middle ear infections.

- Even newborns can be fitted with hearing aids.

- Dizziness is an important *early* warning sign of inner ear damage.

- Hearing loss can be caused by growths and tumors.

- Some scientists believe that allergies may contribute to Ménière's disease, a common cause of hearing loss in women age 35 to 55.

- Occupation is the most common cause of noise-induced hearing loss.

- Noises that are safe for one person may be hazardous for another person.

- Contrary to stereotypes, persons with certain kinds of hearing loss speak too *softly*.

Don't let hearing loss restrict your life. Everything you need to know about the latest therapies, surgical techniques, and assistive devices—including hearing aids, implants, communication enhancers, support groups, and the developing social and workplace rights associated with hearing impairment and hearing-loss prevention—are right here, in this practical, informative, and easy-to-use guide.

WHAT YOU CAN DO ABOUT HEARING LOSS

THE DELL MEDICAL LIBRARY

LEARNING TO LIVE WITH CHRONIC FATIGUE SYNDROME

LEARNING TO LIVE WITH CHRONIC IBS

RELIEF FROM CARPAL TUNNEL SYNDROME AND OTHER REPETITIVE
MOTION DISORDERS

RELIEF FROM HAY FEVER AND OTHER AIRBORNE ALLERGIES

RELIEF FROM CHRONIC ARTHRITIS PAIN

RELIEF FROM CHRONIC BACKACHE

RELIEF FROM CHRONIC HEADACHE

RELIEF FROM CHRONIC HEMORRHOIDS

WHAT YOU CAN DO ABOUT SINUSITIS

RELIEF FROM CHRONIC TMJ PAIN

RELIEF FROM PMS

RELIEF FROM SLEEPING DISORDERS

WHAT WOMEN CAN DO ABOUT CHRONIC ENDOMETRIOSIS

WHAT YOU CAN DO ABOUT ANEMIA

WHAT YOU CAN DO ABOUT BLADDER CONTROL

WHAT YOU CAN DO ABOUT CHRONIC HAIR LOSS

WHAT YOU CAN DO ABOUT CHRONIC SKIN PROBLEMS

WHAT YOU CAN DO ABOUT OSTEOPOROSIS

WHAT WOMEN SHOULD KNOW ABOUT CHRONIC INFECTIONS AND
SEXUALLY TRANSMITTED DISEASES

WHAT WOMEN SHOULD KNOW ABOUT MENOPAUSE

WHAT YOU CAN DO ABOUT ASTHMA

WHAT YOU CAN DO ABOUT DIABETES

WHAT YOU CAN DO ABOUT EATING DISORDERS

WHAT YOU CAN DO ABOUT EPILEPSY

WHAT YOU CAN DO ABOUT INFERTILITY

WHAT YOU CAN DO ABOUT HEARING LOSS

THE DELL MEDICAL LIBRARY

What You Can Do About
HEARING LOSS

Norra Tannenhaus

Foreword by John W. House, M.D.

A LYNN SONBERG BOOK

Published by
Dell Publishing
a division of
Bantam Doubleday Dell Publishing Group, Inc.
1540 Broadway
New York, New York 10036

Research about hearing loss is constantly evolving. While the author has made every effort to include the most accurate and up-to-date information in this book, there can be no guarantee that what we know about this complex subject won't change with time. Please keep in mind that this book is not intended for the purpose of self-diagnosis or self-treatment. The reader should consult his or her physician regarding a suspected hearing problem or any other health concern.

ISBN: 0-440-21656-7

Published by arrangement with Lynn Sonberg Book Services, 260 West 72 Street, 6-C, New York, NY 10023

Printed in the United States of America

Published simultaneously in Canada

October 1993

10 9 8 7 6 5 4 3 2 1
OPM

FOREWORD

Hearing impairments are among the most common medical conditions in the United States today. What's more, their prevalence will grow in the years ahead, as increasing numbers of people live into old age—people who most likely spent some portion of their youth listening to loud rock music or engaging in other activities in which they were exposed to noise.

Fortunately, scientists have noted the rising occurrence of hearing loss and, in the last several decades, have made more progress in hearing research than in perhaps all the years going back to Hippocrates combined. Thanks to these efforts, hearing-impaired people—including those who are completely deaf—are able to lead productive, independent lives.

Nor has science been the only arena for progress. Special schools (including at least one university—Gallaudet University, in Washington, D.C.—geared solely to the needs of deaf students), support groups, and lobbying organizations have made known the needs of hearing-impaired people, with the result that now many classrooms, theaters, houses of worship, televisions, and telephones are equipped to meet the requirements of someone whose hearing is damaged. And as new legislation is passed that protects the rights of all disabled people, the hearing-impaired person's ability to function normally in the world can only grow.

One way to avail yourself of all your options is to learn as much as possible about hearing and hearing loss in general and the nature of your hearing loss in particular. The role of a book such as this is to introduce the hearing-impaired person and those closest to him or her to the basic processes of hearing and what happens when something goes wrong. You'll also discover just how widespread hearing loss really is—how it cuts across all of society, regardless of age, race, or gender. In addition, the book describes some of the remedies available to you and where you can find more information.

But I think the most important section of the book concerns the emotional impact of hearing loss. The biggest problem that we see at the House Ear Clinic occurs when patients deny they have a hearing loss. They may rationalize it by saying that other people mumble, that they don't speak clearly, or similar excuses. If these patients don't face the truth, they can make the problem worse for their family and friends. Often, they withdraw from social contact, because communication with others just becomes too difficult.

I have devoted my life to helping people face their hearing loss and get help for it. One way to acknowledge a hearing loss is to learn more about it—and what better way to do it than by reading this book? Think of it as a friendly guide that explains the basics in simple language and offers suggestions for finding more in-depth information. This is meant to be not a comprehensive text but a good, basic primer to keep by your side.

JOHN W. HOUSE, M.D.
President, House Ear Clinic, Inc.
Associate Clinical Professor of Otolaryngology,
University of Southern California School of Medicine

CONTENTS

Introduction   xi

1   HOW YOU HEAR   1

2   TYPES OF HEARING LOSS   16

3   TESTING AND DIAGNOSING HEARING LOSS   29

4   PREVENTING HEARING LOSS   57

5   COPING WITH HEARING LOSS   75

6   HEARING AIDS, OTHER DEVICES,
    AND SURGERY   94

7   FOR MORE HELP   119

    Glossary   130

    Index   136

    About the Author   142

INTRODUCTION

What happens when you tell someone you're reading a book about hearing loss? There's a good chance he'll lean closer, cup his ear, and say, "Eh? Whad'ya say?" Or something he's sure is equally witty.

But if you're reading this book because you're concerned about yourself or a loved one, you know that hearing loss is no joke. The fact is, there are about 28 million hearing-impaired people in North America, at least 16 million of them in the United States alone. Currently, some 2 million Americans are either totally deaf or so hearing impaired that they cannot hear a normal conversation, a telephone ringing, traffic noise, or a fire alarm. Hearing is moderately to severely impaired in the remaining 14 million people. Each year, doctors report more than 2.1 million new cases of hearing impairment. Globally, it's been estimated that roughly 10 percent *of all the people in the world* have some degree of hearing loss. And that doesn't take into account the people who have to live and work with these individuals—they, too, are affected.

Who *are* all these people? As you might have guessed, hearing loss is most common among the elderly. More than one out of every four people over age 65 has a hearing disorder of some kind. By age 75, hearing loss afflicts substantially more than one out of three.

But hearing loss isn't exclusive to the elderly. It's been estimated that 3 percent of all schoolchildren are affected by hearing impairments, including at least 200,000 children who were either born deaf or suffered a severe hearing loss during the first year or two of life. Some 33 percent of children experience temporary hearing loss due to repeated middle ear infections. And as you'll see in this book, hearing impairments can strike young or middle-aged adults as well, often in the form of noise-induced hearing loss or conditions such as otosclerosis or Ménière's disease, which are described in this book.

What's more, as greater numbers of premature infants (many of whom are born with hearing impairments) survive, as our fondness for rock music and noisy appliances continues unabated, and as more and more of us live into old age, hearing loss will become increasingly common. Some researchers claim that virtually anyone who lives long enough in American society will develop some degree of hearing loss.

So if you have a hearing loss, or know someone who does, you're far from alone—in fact, you're affected by one of the most common ailments known. This doesn't, of course, make a hearing loss any easier to live with, but it does mean that there's a lot of help available. Surgery, hearing aids, devices that help with everyday life, support groups, organizations for advocacy and research, even dogs specially trained to help the hearing impaired—all have been developed to meet the needs of people with a hearing loss and those who care about them.

This book is designed to help you understand more about hearing and hearing loss. It will explain the basic aspects of normal hearing, what can go wrong, and the help that's available to you. Chapter One concentrates on how you hear: the different structures of the ear that make hearing possible and how they interact with sound waves. You'll also learn a bit about the most important characteristics of sound—sound waves, frequency, and volume—and how your ears and brain respond to them to enable you to hear myriads of sounds.

From here, you can go on to Chapter Two, which describes different types of hearing loss. You'll learn in more detail what can go wrong in the hearing process and how that can result in different types of impairment.

For people who *do* show signs of hearing loss, in Chapter Three we'll offer tips for finding a hearing specialist. We'll also describe the tests your doctor or audiologist will be most likely to perform, as well as some of the conditions he or she will probably suspect.

In Chapter Four, we'll delve further into the main causes of hearing loss. Noise-induced hearing loss is by far the most common cause of hearing loss in the United States, and in separate sections, you'll discover how noise does its damage and how you can protect yourself from it.

The first step in getting help for a hearing impairment is to acknowledge that the impairment exists. Some people have no problem with that, but many others do. A lot of people equate hearing loss with old age, senility, or loss of prowess or mental faculties; others may be embarrassed or afraid or simply don't want to admit that their bodies may not be working perfectly anymore. Denial not only diminishes the quality of their own lives; it affects the people who must live or work with them. Chapter Five deals with the emotional impact of hearing loss: how it can affect the person's life and relationships with family, coworkers, and friends and how it may perpetuate a vicious cycle of loneliness, helplessness, and isolation. If you're reading this book out of concern for someone with a hearing loss, you'll learn what you can do to improve communication and encourage that person to seek help.

It's ironic that so many people allow hearing loss to isolate or embarrass them because hearing loss *is* such a common condition. More important, it's *treatable*. Doctors have made enormous advances in surgical techniques in the last 30 to 40 years, including developing and refining cochlear implants, which can help people whose hearing nerves no longer function. Chapter Six describes a number of medical interventions—surgical and nonsurgical—readily available to treat hearing loss.

Essentially, then, this book contains basic descriptions of normal ear function, what goes wrong, what to expect from medical experts, how to cope emotionally, and some idea of what kind of help is available. But so much is going on in the field of hearing loss research that it's impossible to include it all in a book such as this. However, we *can* tell you how to find more information if you're interested, and Chapter Seven does precisely that. There are dozens, perhaps hundreds, of organizations devoted to all facets of the problem of hearing loss—support groups, research organizations, special schools, professional societies, and so on. If you want more information on any subject related to hearing impairment, chances are you'll find it through at least one of the organizations listed here.

Finally, there's a glossary for quick reference to the medical terminology used throughout the book.

* * *

Remember: Hearing loss affects virtually everyone—if not directly, then indirectly by striking a loved one, friend, or colleague. And while doctors still can't always restore hearing to normal, there's much that they *can* do to ensure that your life will remain normal nonetheless. You've only to learn more about the causes of hearing loss and the best methods of coping with them. And there's no better way to begin than by reading this book.

HOW YOU HEAR

Your ears play an obvious role in helping you stay in touch with your world. You can hear your baby cry, an alarm go off, your boss's instructions, the whistle of an oncoming train. You can enjoy a Beethoven symphony or a Top 40 tune; you can hear birds sing, dogs bark, lions roar.

But good hearing plays a more subtle role as well. Some sounds are there even if you're not actually listening to them—they hover on the edge of perception. An air conditioner hums; traffic goes by; there are voices in the hall. Your kids are watching television in the next room; someone is running water; your cat is eating the dry food you've left out for him. Perhaps a neighbor's telephone rings, or maybe you have a grandfather clock whose hourly chiming you don't even hear anymore. Yet something would be missing without these sounds. We live in a virtual ocean of sound, and without it, the world can seem a bleak place indeed.

The organs that let us perceive all this are finely tuned instruments, at once easily damaged yet remarkably tough. Enclosed within a few inches on either side of the skull, the ears, when functioning well, let us hear everything from the slightest whisper to cannon fire. And hearing isn't the only job our ears perform; they also help maintain our sense of balance and the correct pressure in the middle ear and throat.

To understand how the ears accomplish all this, and to understand what can go wrong when we start losing our hearing, we first have to learn a little about ear structure and function.

EAR ANATOMY

The sense of hearing develops surprisingly early in life. Some experiments indicate that a fetus in its mother's womb may detect certain kinds of sound at around 26 weeks of gestation.

In adults, the ears reside in the *temporal bone,* the hardest bone in the body. Doctors divide the ear into three basic parts: the outer ear, the middle ear, and the inner ear. A problem in any or all of these areas may lead to a hearing loss, but your chances of having your hearing restored depend heavily on the cause of the impairment and the part of the ear affected.

The Outer Ear

The external, or outer, ear has two components. The first is that part of the ear you actually see—those curved structures attached to either side of your head. This part of the ear is called the *auricle,* or *pinna.* It is composed primarily of cartilage and skin.

The main function of the pinna is to direct sound waves into the second portion of the outer ear, the *ear canal*. This tiny canal, about one-fourth inch around, extends about one inch into the head and leads directly to the eardrum. During its brief journey, the canal narrows a little in the middle, then widens again, giving it something of an hourglass shape. The ear canal contains glands that produce earwax, or *cerumen*, and also contains hair. Together the hair and wax protect the eardrum from dust, from other airborne particles, and even from insects; the wax also contains a chemical that kills bacteria, thus guarding against infection. As far as hearing is concerned, the ear canal acts as a resonating chamber and enhances the volume of some of the sounds necessary for understanding speech.

The Middle Ear

The eardrum, also called the *tympanum* or *tympanic membrane,* forms the boundary between the outer and middle ear. This thin, exquisitely sensitive membrane, roughly the diameter of the eraser on a pencil, stretches across the ear canal and, like a drum, vibrates when sound waves bounce against it. These vibrations are then transmitted to the next middle ear component, three minuscule bones known collectively as the *ossicles.*

Many people remember this part of ear anatomy from their grade-school science classes because the individual ossicles have such quaint names: the *hammer,* the *anvil,* and the *stirrup.* One side of the hammer presses right up against the eardrum; the other side contacts the anvil, which in turn touches the stirrup. Thus, when the eardrum vibrates, the ossicles also vibrate in turn. By compressing or concentrating the sound wave as it travels through the ear, these three tiny bones, packed into a space roughly the size of an aspirin, amplify the vibrations so that they don't fade away before you're actually able to perceive the sound.

The final bone in this sequence, the stirrup, is the smallest bone in your body. As it vibrates, the stirrup strikes a membrane known as the *oval window*, which marks the transition from middle to inner ear. Thus, the stirrup plays a crucial role in the transmission of sound through the ear; if it doesn't vibrate freely against the oval window, your hearing may be impaired. And as you'll see in the next chapter, this is in fact a common cause of hearing loss.

The Inner Ear

The oval window divides the middle from the inner ear. It moves in response to vibrations from the stirrup and, in turn, transmits these vibrations to the base of a structure known as the *cochlea*.

Roughly the size of a pea, the snail-shaped cochlea contains the organ of Corti, the component that's responsible for transmitting sound waves to the brain, which interprets them into the sounds that we actually perceive. On the organ of Corti are cells known as *hair cells* because they resemble hairs when seen under a microscope; these are the cells that actually detect the sound waves and transmit the message to the brain.

The cochlea also contains fluid. When the oval window vibrates against the base of the cochlea, it causes waves or

Ear anatomy

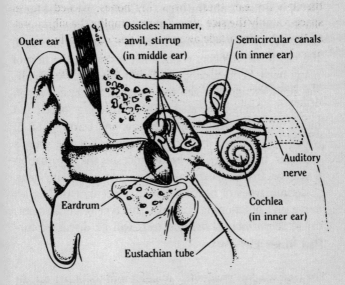

vibrations within the fluid. Since this liquid bathes the organ of Corti, when it moves, the hair cells move with it. Nerve fibers in contact with the hair cells detect this motion, and respond by sending nerve impulses to the brain. This is what permits you to hear and interpret the sounds around you.

The semicircular canals, loop-shaped tubular structures, are also located in the inner ear and are responsible for balance.

The Auditory Nerve

Nerve impulses from the organ of Corti travel to the brain via the auditory nerve, also called the *eighth cranial nerve* or simply the *eighth nerve.* Soon after entering the brain, the eighth nerve fibers contact nerve cells in the first of many nerve centers concerned with hearing. Ultimately, the auditory signals reach the cortex of the brain, which contains centers associated with interpreting speech and music, as well as thinking, memory, and learning, all of which are involved in helping you interpret the sounds you hear. In this way, the brain processes the information it receives from the ears into the sound you actually hear.

Certain types of hearing loss may occur if the eighth nerve isn't functioning properly. This type of impairment, called *sensorineural hearing loss,* will be discussed further in Chapter Two.

In summary, then, the external ear conducts sound waves into the ear canal, where they strike the eardrum and cause it to vibrate. These vibrations are transmitted through the middle ear by the hammer, anvil, and stirrup; the stirrup then sends its vibrations into the fluid of the cochlea, where hair cells on the organ of Corti convert the vibrations into nerve impulses that travel to the brain along the auditory nerve.

The middle and inner ear contain other structures, which help maintain balance and equalize pressure. They'll be covered in more detail toward the end of this chapter. Before that, let's take a closer look at the nature of sound.

SOUND WAVES

For a clearer understanding of what goes wrong in various kinds of hearing problems, it's important to have a rudimentary knowledge of sound waves and how we perceive them.

Sound waves cause molecules in the air to vibrate. For example, when you speak, air rushes through your vocal cords and makes them reverberate. This, in turn, causes molecules in the surrounding air to vibrate and collide with one another, thus setting in motion the sound waves that hit the eardrum and eventually permit everyone to hear what you have to say. The outer ear conducts the sound waves to the middle ear; the middle ear transforms the airborne vibrations into waves in the fluid of the cochlea; and the inner ear receives these messages and sends them along to the brain.

It's important to remember that until all these steps have occurred and the sound message has reached the brain, *you haven't heard a thing.* So if the signal is weakened or distorted at any point, your perception of it—that is, your hearing—will be impaired.

The Spectrum of Sound

Just as light is composed of a whole spectrum of colors, sound is made up of a range of frequencies—from extremely low, below the lowest note on a bass fiddle, to very high, above the highest note on a piccolo. A sound's pitch depends on its frequency: A high-pitched sound is a high-frequency sound, and a low-pitched sound is a low-frequency sound. In physiological terms, a high-pitched vibration pushes against the eardrum, whereas a low-pitched vibration pulls the eardrum forward. The hair cells on the organ of Corti are specialized to respond to sound vibrations of different frequencies.

In general, vowels are low-frequency sounds. Strong and easily heard, vowel sounds travel well across rooms and around corners. It's also relatively easy to hear vowel sounds over background noise. Consonants, on the other hand, are weaker, higher-frequency sounds. They don't hold up well over a distance and tend to get lost if someone speaks to you from around a corner or in a noisy room.

The Vocabulary of Sound

A scientist might describe *frequency* as "the number of cycles per second at which a particular sound travels through air or water." A *cycle* is composed of one high-pitched sound vibration and one corresponding low-pitched vibration. That's why you'll often see frequency measured in units called *cycles per second,* or *cps.* These units may also be referred to as *Hertz,* or *Hz.* Human ears can't detect anything much lower than about 20 Hz or higher than around 20,000 Hz. Our ears seem to be most sensitive within the range of 1,000 to 4,000 Hz. That means we can detect sounds in these frequencies at a volume lower than what would be needed to hear sounds outside this frequency range.

Usually, hearing loss occurs in the higher frequencies first. Thus, people with hearing loss often have a lot of trouble hearing consonants or diphthongs such as *s, sh, th,* or *f.* Other consonant sounds like *p* and *t* may sound too much alike, making a hearing-impaired person mistake one for the other.

People sometimes confuse *frequency* with *volume*. *Frequency* refers to a sound's pitch, whereas *volume* refers to its loudness. Volume is measured in units called *decibels,* or *db.* The volume threshold at which most healthy young adults can start to hear anything is considered 0 db; 20 db is the volume of an average whisper. Most people can hear a conversation comfortably at 65 to 70 db; anything louder than 85 db is considered potentially hazardous to the ears. The difference between 65 db and 85 db may not seem like much, but consider this: A sound that is 10 db greater than another sound is 10 times louder; if it's 20 db greater, it's 100 times louder; 30 db greater, 1,000 times louder; and so on. Thus, an 85-db sound is *100 times louder* than a sound that's only 65 db.

Binaural Hearing

Binaural hearing refers to the fact that we normally hear with two ears. A sound reaches the ear closer to it a split second before it reaches the other ear. This happens too quickly for you to be aware of it, but that infinitesimal fraction of a second is enough time for the brain to interpret the two signals and let you determine where the sound is coming from. If the hearing in one ear is impaired more than in the other, it can affect your ability to locate sounds.

THE OTHER FUNCTIONS OF THE EAR

Most people know that that popping sensation they feel when descending from a great height has something to do with the middle ear. In fact, that feeling results when a middle ear component called the *eustachian tube* tries to equalize the air pressure in the middle ear, on either side of the eardrum.

In its brief span of one and a half inches, the eustachian tube connects the middle ear to the *nasopharynx,* that part of the throat behind the nasal passages. One end of the tube opens into the middle ear cavity; the other, into the back of the throat. When functioning properly, the eustachian tube opens for a fraction of a second roughly once every three minutes in response to a swallow or a yawn. This allows air into the middle ear to replace air that's been absorbed by the tissues lining the middle ear or to equalize pressure changes that occur due to changes in altitude. Anything that interferes with this periodic opening and closing of the eustachian tube may impair hearing, because the middle ear requires an air-filled environment for the ossicles to vibrate properly.

Why do your ears hurt during an airplane's descent? Sometimes the eustachian tube stays closed, which means it can't maintain equal pressure on both sides of the eardrum. As a result, pressure builds up on the outer side of the eardrum, forcing it to bulge into the middle ear cavity and leading to the sensation of pain. That's why people tell you to yawn, swallow, or chew gum: All these activities encourage the eustachian tube to open.

Have you been told to avoid flying if you have a cold? That's because a cold or an allergy may block the eustachian tube, which can also impair its function. In fact, many hearing-impaired people report that their hearing gets even worse for a while following a plane flight, possibly because their eustachian tubes don't function normally.

Thus, while the eustachian tube isn't directly involved in the process of hearing, it does help maintain good hearing by promoting an environment in which the middle ear can function properly.

Balancing Act

The cochlea isn't the only fluid-filled organ in the inner ear. Connected to the cochlea are the semicircular canals, which, like the cochlea, contain fluid—actually, it's more of a jellylike substance—and hair cells. And as in the cochlea, the hair cells move in response to motions in the liquid. Only this liquid doesn't respond to sound waves. Instead, it moves whenever you change the position of your head. For example, if you stand up, close your eyes, and shake your head no, you'll be able to keep your balance, because your brain uses the information it receives and interprets from the hair cells in different areas of the semicircular canals. The action of the jellylike fluid in the semicircular canals helps you perceive your body's position and stay level, even when your eyes are closed. People with ear infections sometimes complain of feeling dizzy because the infection may have spread into their semicircular canals.

DOCTOR, I FEEL DIZZY!

Hearing loss isn't the only signal that something may be awry with one or both ears. Dizziness, with or without hearing loss, is another tip-off that inner ear function may be damaged. However, hearing-impaired people do experience balance problems more often than the general population because the mechanisms controlling balance are located in the inner ear. This organ is so small, and its structures so close together, that an injury or disease is rarely confined to one portion only.

As mentioned earlier, the inner ear helps you maintain your balance, in addition to the role it plays in hearing. The vestibular apparatus and semicircular canals, which are attached to the cochlea, work in concert with the eyes so that you adjust quickly and easily to sudden changes in movement or position. The normal function of this ear–eye system, called the vestibuloocular system, is to coordinate your eye movements with those changes. When you move your head or turn around rapidly, your eyes go through a characteristic series of movements known as *nystagmus*. If that coordination is disrupted, you feel dizzy.

Sometimes dizziness is a normal reaction, such as when you turn around in circles for a moment or two. In these cases, the dizziness should resolve on its own a few minutes after you stop spinning. But in other cases, people feel dizzy even when they're sitting or lying perfectly still. For example, if the vestibular apparatus in someone's left ear has been damaged for some reason, he may have the sensation that his head is always turning right, and he'll try to adjust his eye movements accordingly. This person may even feel as if he's continually falling to the left, and this feeling may intensify when he closes his eyes. And remember, all these sensations may occur while the individual is actually sitting still, so his discomfort can be considerable.

Dizziness has several causes and may take different forms. The treatment will depend on the diagnosis your doctor makes and what he or she thinks is the reason for the condition.

Vertigo

Defined as the sensation of motion (one doctor refers to it as a "hallucination" of motion, because you aren't really moving), *vertigo* is perhaps the most common form of dizziness associated with inner ear dysfunction or disease. People may say they feel as if they're rocking, tilting, or spinning. Interestingly, doctors often find that the more severe the vertigo, the less serious the cause.

The most common cause of vertigo is a condition known as *benign paroxysmal positional vertigo,* or *BPPV,* in which people feel dizzy when they're lying down. Doctors aren't sure what initiates BPPV, but it seems to resolve on its own, with no permanent damage. Until it goes away, the person affected can do special exercises to relieve the dizzy feeling. Among the other possible causes of vertigo are anything that injures the appropriate inner ear structures, some drugs, tumors of the eighth nerve or some areas of the brain, or Ménière's disease, a condition resulting from fluid buildup in the inner ear.

WHAT GOES WRONG?

As you've seen, hearing is a complicated process that consists of lots of steps and requires many small, delicate structures. And as you might have guessed, the causes of hearing loss are almost as numerous as all the different factors involved. This chapter will end with an overview of the major kinds of hearing loss, which will be covered in more detail in Chapter Two.

Hearing loss may arise from a problem anywhere in the outer, middle, or inner ear. When the outer ear is affected, it's usually from some kind of blockage in the ear canal. Earwax often accumulates and may form a plug that sometimes gets pushed up against the eardrum, which prevents it from reverberating in response to sound waves, with obvious effects on hearing. It's also not unusual for small children to get foreign objects stuck in their ears, with the same results. Foreign objects occasionally also become lodged in adults' ear canals. There are even a few horrific cases on record in medical journals in which insects have managed to crawl into people's ears! (Hearing was restored to normal after doctors killed and removed the bugs.) Infections of the ear canal, known as *otitis externa,* may also affect hearing.

In the middle ear, hearing loss usually results from damage to the eardrum or the ossicles. Damage may be caused by a middle ear infection (*otitis media*); by fluid in the middle ear (*serous otitis media,* perhaps the most common cause of middle ear impairment); or by a fairly common condition called *otosclerosis,* in which the stirrup can no longer vibrate freely in response to the movements of the hammer and anvil.

There are many conditions that affect the inner ear and

lead to hearing loss. Middle ear infections that spread to the inner ear, medical problems such as hardening of the arteries (which may affect circulation in the ear), or specific diseases such as Ménière's disease (which affects the cochlea and semicircular canals) are just a few of the things that can go wrong in this part of the ear.

Fortunately, doctors have made enormous strides in the treatment of hearing loss. If the hearing problem experienced by you or a loved one is centered in the outer or middle ear, chances are good that your hearing can be restored to normal or nearly normal. Inner ear hearing losses, alas, have as yet eluded most attempts at treatment, but a virtually endless array of assistive devices can help you cope with just about every conceivable aspect of living. However, to use any treatment or device to its fullest advantage, you must have the clearest possible picture of your condition—its causes, the parts of the ear affected, how to manage it, and how to prevent your hearing from getting any worse. Chapters Two and Three look at what can go wrong in the hearing process, how doctors evaluate your hearing, and how they can help you cope with a hearing loss.

TYPES OF
HEARING LOSS

Different types of hearing loss may be identified by degree
—mild, moderate, severe, or profound—or by the nature
of the impairment—conductive, sensorineural, or mixed.
This short chapter will explain the differences among the
various types of hearing loss, so you can better understand the testing procedures and conditions described in
Chapter Three.

DEGREES OF HEARING IMPAIRMENT

In general, doctors and other professionals who specialize
in the field of hearing and speech disorders group hearing
loss into four very general categories, according to the
severity of the problem.

Mild Hearing Loss

People are said to have a mild hearing loss when they can hear strong, low-frequency sounds, like vowels in speech, but not weaker, higher-frequency sounds, such as consonants.

Moderate Hearing Loss

As the name implies, this type of hearing loss occurs in the midfrequency ranges.

Severe Hearing Loss

Severe hearing loss is usually defined as the inability to hear sounds at 65 to 90 db of volume. In general, normal conversation occurs at around 60 to 70 db. Thus, the practical meaning of a severe hearing loss is that you can no longer hear most conversation.

Profound Hearing Loss

People with a profound hearing loss have almost completely lost the ability to hear. They require lessons in speech (lip) reading, as well as powerful hearing aids and other assistive devices.

TYPES OF HEARING LOSS

As you saw in Chapter One, hearing is a complicated process, involving many steps and many intricate mechanisms. A problem anywhere along the way can affect your ability to hear.

However, while the outcome of all these problems may be the same—hearing loss—the point at which the problems occur determines the nature and the degree of the hearing loss and your doctor's ability to treat it. For these reasons, the different kinds of hearing loss are usually identified according to the anatomic structures involved.

Conductive Hearing Loss

A conductive hearing loss involves an impairment of the outer or middle ear. This type of hearing loss is described as "conductive" because it occurs during the early steps of the hearing process, in which sound is picked up and conducted from the outer into the middle and inner ear. Usually, it means that sounds can't reach the inner ear properly because there's something blocking the pathway through the outer or middle ear. The result is that you can still hear everything, but it all sounds muffled. You might be able to simulate this feeling by stuffing cotton in your ears or simply holding your outer ears closed with your fingers. People with conductive hearing losses may also experience ear pain or discharge. In general, the hearing loss is mild, which means it occurs around 60 db or above. Thus, people with conductive hearing losses can still hear some speech or other sounds if they're loud enough; these individuals also derive maximum benefit from hearing aids.

Causes of Conductive Hearing Loss. What causes conductive hearing loss? Usually, there's an obstruction of some kind in the ear canal, damage to the eardrum, or a middle ear infection.

Obstruction in the ear canal. Impacted earwax is the most common cause of obstruction. Normally, earwax is soft. Produced by glands within the ear canal, it usually just falls out of the ear when it's served its purpose. But in some people, the wax becomes hard and builds up to form a plug, which may in time completely block the ear canal, preventing sound waves from reaching the eardrum. Usually, your hearing isn't affected until the blockage is total.

One of the symptoms of earwax impaction is a sudden, dramatic decrease in hearing; thus, you shouldn't be alarmed if you experience this, because it doesn't necessarily indicate a serious problem, but do see a doctor as soon as you can. If you do have impacted earwax, it should be removed by your family doctor or an *otologist* (a doctor who specializes in diseases of the ear) to prevent damage to the skin lining the ear canal. Attempts at cleaning your ear yourself, with a finger, a tissue, or a cotton swab, may only pack the earwax more firmly and may even damage the eardrum if you press hard enough. Many hearing specialists tell their patients, "Never put anything smaller than your elbow in your ear." Some people find over-the-counter earwax-softening preparations helpful, but others have an allergic reaction to them. It's best to let your doctor recommend the right product for you.

It's not uncommon for earwax blockage to occur after

swimming, because the wax plug may absorb some water and swell. People who swim a lot may also develop bony growths in the ear canal, which may in turn promote more wax accumulation. If you experience a persistent hearing loss after swimming, see your doctor and, again, have him or her remove any accumulation of earwax.

As you've probably guessed, *anything* that blocks the ear canal can lead to a conductive hearing loss. Small children are notoriously prone to stuffing odd things, like corn kernels or peanuts, in their ears, then forgetting about them until they're reminded by loss of hearing, ear pain, or an ear discharge. Once again, any foreign object should be removed by a professional.

In adults, eczema or *dermatitis* (irritation of the skin) often occurs in the ear canal. Vigorous scratching may break the skin, leaving it open to infection and swelling, with the end result of blocking the ear canal and causing a conductive hearing loss. As with all the conditions discussed here, this should be checked by a doctor, but if the symptoms are mild, many physicians simply recommend an over-the-counter cortisone cream to relieve the itching and discourage scratching.

Middle ear infection. Among problems in the middle ear, the most common cause by far of conductive hearing loss is *otitis media,* or middle ear infection. Children are the most common victims of otitis media, but adults can get it, too; germs from any bad cold, allergy, or other form of upper respiratory tract infection may travel from the nasal sinuses through the eustachian tube into the middle ear. Often, this results from holding both nostrils closed while blowing your nose, which forces mucus, and the germs it contains, into the eustachian tube. A safer way to blow your nose, especially when you're ill, is to press lightly on one nostril at a time and blow gently.

Ear pain is usually the first symptom of a middle ear infection, especially if it develops in conjunction with a cold or an allergy attack. The infection causes fluid buildup in the middle ear, leading to pressure against the inner surface of the eardrum, which causes the pain. Hearing loss may result because the eardrum and/or middle ear bones can no longer vibrate freely in response to sound. For a more detailed discussion of otitis media as a cause of hearing loss, see Chapter Four.

Eardrum damage. A perforated eardrum is another common cause of conductive hearing loss. This problem occurs more than you might imagine, and it can be the result of injury, infection, or even a sudden change in atmospheric pressure. Many people wince at the very thought of a hole in the eardrum, but actually, doctors today can repair damaged eardrums fairly easily or even rebuild them completely if necessary.

Congenital anomalies. Finally, conductive hearing losses may arise from genetic or congenital abnormalities (*congenital* means the defect is present from birth, although it's not necessarily related to genetics). For example, the outer or middle ear may be deformed due to hereditary problems or because of an illness or injury that affects the baby at or near the time of birth. Often, doctors can correct these problems with surgery.

Signs of Conductive Hearing Loss. How do you know if you or someone close to you has a conductive hearing impairment? The symptoms include:

Speaking too softly. A conductive hearing loss doesn't affect the inner ear. Therefore, individuals with this problem won't hear other people's voices that well but will perceive their own voices as being louder than the voices of those around them. To compensate, they lower their own voices to a volume they believe comparable with everyone else's.

Hearing voices better in noisy surroundings than when it's quiet. At a loud restaurant or a rowdy party, people naturally have to raise their voices if they want to be heard by anybody. This makes it easier for the person with a conductive hearing impairment to hear them, in spite of the background noise. It may even be *because of* the background noise; some scientists think that continuous background noise may somehow render the ears' conductive mechanisms more sensitive to speech. There's also the possibility that hearing-impaired people have unconsciously learned to do a little lipreading.

The ability to tolerate noises that would be too loud for people with normal hearing and painfully loud for those with other types of hearing loss. Again, this is because the outer and middle ears can't conduct sound to the inner ear.

Hearing better through bone, rather than air, conduction. The entire ear mechanism resides in a bone called the *mastoid bone*, which is part of a larger structure called the *temporal bone*. Certain sounds can make the mastoid bone vibrate, which in turn leads to vibrations in the cochlea fluid and culminates in the perception of those sounds, in much the same way that sound coming through the ear canal also causes the cochlea fluid to vibrate. For example, if you press your ear against a vibrating surface, you may be able to detect sound that's transmitted through the bone, sometimes even if it's too faint to be heard through the air. When we speak, we hear our own voices through both air *and* bone conduction, but when we listen to ourselves on a recording, we hear mostly via air conduction—that's why it's such a shock when you hear your recorded voice for the first time. If you have a conductive hearing loss, you'll hear better when sounds are conducted through the bone rather than through the air because airborne sounds require functioning outer and middle ears to be heard properly.

The good news about conductive hearing impairments is that most of them can be repaired with medical and/or surgical intervention; in fact, doctors can often restore hearing to normal in these cases. And even if someone's conductive hearing loss can't be completely reversed, his or her chances of using, and adapting well to, a hearing aid are excellent.

Sensorineural Hearing Loss

Problems in the inner ear lead to a type of impairment known as sensorineural hearing loss and involve damage either to the ear's *sensory* components (such as the hair cells in the cochlea, or other parts of the inner ear) or to the *neural* components of hearing (the eighth nerve or the hearing centers in the brain). The end result of this type of damage is that the inner ear can no longer transmit sound to the brain. Because nerve impairment is often an important part of this phenomenon, sensorineural hearing loss is also referred to as *nerve deafness*.

Causes of Sensorineural Hearing Loss

Noise.   Noise is the most common culprit—especially if you're exposed to it on the job, eight hours a day, five days a week, 50 weeks a year, for several years at a stretch. You'll learn more about noise-induced hearing loss in Chapter Four, but for now, rest assured that if this is your problem, you share it with tens of millions of people around the world.

Head injuries.   Accidents, strokes, hemorrhaging in the brain, or even a strong blow to the head—any of these may damage the inner ear and/or the brain areas responsible for hearing and may lead to nerve deafness.

Age-related problems.   Hearing loss related to aging, known as *presbycusis*, is another form of sensorineural hearing loss. At the other end of the age spectrum, most congenital hearing problems also lead to nerve deafness, although there are those few that are associated with conductive impairments. Hearing loss at birth may be the outcome of an especially difficult labor and delivery, or it may be contracted by the developing fetus if the mother catches a viral infection, like measles, German measles, or mumps. That's why it's so important for women to be vaccinated against these infections *before* they become pregnant: They're protecting the health of their future offspring, as well as their own well-being. Indeed, these same infections may damage the hair cells of the cochlea in adults and lead to hearing loss in them as well. If you've recently suffered a bout of any of these disorders, or the flu, scarlet fever, or meningitis, have your hearing checked even if the disease has been cured. (Interestingly, the middle and outer ear infections described in the previous sections rarely lead to sensorineural hearing loss.)

Tumors of the eighth nerve. These benign tumors are yet another cause of nerve deafness. They may actually grow between the cochlea and the eighth nerve, pressing on the nerve and ultimately disrupting its function. Usually, the tumors affect only one ear, but there have been cases in which they've been found in both ears. Often, hearing loss is the first sign that the growth—called an *acoustic neuroma*—exists.

If the acoustic neuroma is detected and removed early in its course, recovery from its effects is usually complete. If not treated until later on, the tumor may cause permanent hearing and balance problems or facial paralysis; in some cases, it may even be life-threatening. The symptoms of acoustic neuroma include hearing loss in one or both ears, dizziness, *tinnitus* (ringing or buzzing in the ear), and a feeling of numbness in the face. If these sound like the symptoms of a lot of the ear problems mentioned in this book, you're right—such changes may herald anything from a simple infection to a life-threatening tumor. That's why it's important to see a doctor immediately if you experience any of them.

Prescription drugs. Aspirin, the antibiotics streptomycin and neomycin, and certain kinds of diuretics taken by people who have high blood pressure are all known to damage the hair cells in the inner ear. If you've been taking any of these products—or indeed, any kind of medication—and experience a sudden loss of hearing with or without dizziness or tinnitus, notify your doctor at once. Often, he or she can save you from permanent inner ear damage simply by changing your prescription.

Symptoms of Sensorineural Hearing Loss

Speaking louder than usual.   This is often the first sign of nerve deafness. You may recall that people with a conductive hearing loss may speak more softly than usual because their own voices sound louder to them. With a sensorineural hearing loss, it's just the opposite: Bone conduction doesn't function that well in these individuals; so they can't hear their own voices, and they speak more loudly to compensate. The ability to understand other people's speech may also be impaired, because of the high-frequency deficit that's often one of the earliest signals of nerve deafness. You may still be able to hear vowel sounds, but you won't be able to detect higher-frequency sounds, like consonants. Thus, the words *same, fame,* and *came* may all sound alike—you'll hear the long *a,* but you won't be able to make out the consonants that distinguish these words from each other.

Difficulty hearing speech in noisy places.   Again, this is the opposite of what's seen with conductive hearing loss. In addition, the perception of volume is often abnormal in people with nerve deafness: You may hear fine up to a certain level, at which point your perception of the volume may be completely out of proportion to the sound's actual loudness. In other words, sounds at or above a certain volume level may seem excessively loud to you. Combined with the inability to hear consonants, this makes for impaired hearing and a lot of discomfort in a noisy room.

Changes in pitch perception. Certain tones may seem higher or lower than they really are, or the two ears may differ in the way they hear certain sounds. This even happens with tinnitus, that constant ringing or buzzing in the ears that afflicts so many people. There's evidence that the tinnitus in people with sensorineural hearing loss is higher pitched than in people who have tinnitus for other reasons.

As you might have guessed, sensorineural hearing loss is more difficult to treat than conductive hearing impairment, and there's no guarantee that your hearing will return to normal. Nevertheless, there's a lot that can be done for people with this form of deafness—auditory training (so you can derive maximum understanding from the sounds you do hear); speech retraining (so you can continue to speak clearly); training in sign language, cued speed, and lipreading; and hearing aids and many other types of assistive devices—to permit even the most completely stone-deaf among us to live normally.

Other Types of Hearing Impairments

Mixed Impairment. In some people, the middle ear and inner ear may be affected simultaneously, resulting in a hearing loss that's both conductive *and* sensorineural. For obvious reasons, this is known as a *mixed impairment*.

Central Hearing Loss. Hearing loss may also result from damage to the nerves leading from the inner ear to the brain or from damage to the hearing centers of the brain itself. In either case, this is called *central hearing loss* because it affects the central nervous system. With central hearing loss, the brain misinterprets the hearing signals sent to it. Thus, people with this type of impairment hear the actual sound just fine—their perception of volume and pitch is unaffected. But they can't understand what's being said. Central hearing losses may result from anything that disrupts brain function: a brain tumor; blood vessel damage such as a stroke or cerebral hemorrhage; or injuries such as gunshot wounds, skull fractures, or concussions. Occasionally, a child's head may be injured during an especially difficult delivery; this, too, may result in central deafness if the appropriate areas of the brain are affected.

Most doctors view central hearing impairment as a neurological problem, rather than as a true hearing defect, because it results from damage to the brain and not from problems with any ear structure. Therefore, it falls into the realm of the neurologist, not the hearing specialist.

In this chapter, we've covered the basic ways in which your hearing may become impaired, some possible causes, and some tip-offs that you or a loved one may indeed have a problem. The next step, of course, is to be checked by a doctor. In Chapter Three, you'll learn about the hearing tests you'll most likely undergo and what they mean. Chapter Four describes some of the most common causes of hearing loss. And in the chapters to come, you'll see how much help is available to those who know where to look.

TESTING AND DIAGNOSING HEARING LOSS

Laura rarely went to parties, but she was glad she made herself go to this one. She'd met some fascinating people, a certain man in particular. Upon learning he was Canadian, she asked if he spoke French. She realized he was hard of hearing when he replied, "Oh, yes, I have lots of friends."

On the other side of the room, Frank wasn't having such a good time. Most of the people he tried to make conversation with mumbled unintelligibly, and the music in the background seemed unusually loud and intrusive. As soon as he could politely get away, Frank returned to his home and the book he'd been reading.

Cynthia, on the other hand, was in no condition to go anywhere. Seven months into a difficult pregnancy, she was content just to stay home and watch television. However, lately her husband often complained that the volume was too loud, even though for Cynthia it was just

*right. She began to wonder, "Could there be something
wrong with my hearing?"*

Perhaps you've wondered the same thing about yourself
or someone you know. Maybe you suspect your mom or
dad doesn't hear as well as she or he used to, but you'd
hate to say anything without better evidence. Worse yet,
maybe a few things have happened to you—you've misun-
derstood directions, missed the punch line to a joke, or
seen the look on someone's face when you've answered a
question in a way that clearly didn't make sense. Frank,
mentioned in the second anecdote above, saw some of the
people around him laugh from time to time, but he
couldn't fathom what they were laughing at because he
couldn't hear what was being said. This just added to his
frustration and feelings of awkwardness.

SIGNS OF POSSIBLE HEARING LOSS

There are some telltale signals when someone starts hearing less. Does he or she (or do you):

• Ask people to repeat themselves several times?

• Often appear to be daydreaming or just "not there"?

• Play the radio or television so loudly that companions
  complain about it, or has he or she stopped watching
  or listening entirely?

• Seem to be watching people more carefully as they
  speak?

• Say "Huh?" or "What?" more and more often?

- Avoid strangers or groups of people and resist talking on the telephone?

- Appear lost at parties and other gatherings?

- Misunderstand what's said or sometimes ignore it entirely?

- Seem to have particular trouble understanding someone who speaks rapidly or unexpectedly?

All these are indications of a possible hearing loss. But perhaps the biggest telltale sign is when a formerly sociable person starts withdrawing more and more from contact with others. Imagine how frustrating life becomes for people who can't hear as well as they used to: They can no longer follow the thread of a conversation; perhaps they can't hear movies or plays all that well. Maybe music doesn't sound the way it used to. Or maybe they've been embarrassed too many times when they leave home—strangers can be terribly impatient with people who need a little more time or attention. And if attempts at communication lead to discomfort, arguments, or misunderstanding, who needs it? It's not hard to see why a hearing-impaired person finds it easier simply to withdraw.

Aside from the aforementioned changes in behavior, there are some physical warnings to alert you to a possible hearing loss. These include:

- Pain in, or a discharge from, one or both ears

- Dizziness, especially if there's no apparent cause

- Diminished ability to hear certain tones or certain people's voices, especially if they're high-pitched, like children's voices

- Ringing in the ear (tinnitus)

- Favoring one ear more than the other

- Lack of response to nearby sounds

- A feeling of fullness or discomfort in one or both ears

- Any awareness of a change in hearing

Test Yourself

The American Academy of Otolaryngology—Head and Neck Surgery (AAO-HNS) has devised a simple test for people who may be wondering if they should have their hearing tested. This quiz was field-tested on 71 older patients in five cities; hearing tests were also run on them. Those people whose quiz scores indicated a need to see a physician were confirmed, on the hearing test, as having a hearing impairment.

To take the test, mark the column that best describes the frequency with which you experience each situation or feeling.

Finally, see a doctor *immediately* if you experience (1) a sudden hearing loss or (2) hearing loss accompanied by pain, dizziness, ringing, or roaring in the ear; a feeling of pressure in one or both ears; or ear drainage.

CAN MY CHILD HEAR NORMALLY?

Hearing-impaired children face all the same obstacles as hearing-impaired adults—plus an extra burden: Children must be able to hear others speak so that they can learn to speak normally themselves. And as language is the foundation of learning and social interaction, children's success in school and in life depends heavily on their ability to communicate and to understand others.

Signals of Hearing Impairment

Potential problems are discernible in newborns as well as in older children. Some kinds of hearing loss don't become apparent until a child is a little older; so the fact that a child may have had normal hearing in infancy does not necessarily mean that his or her hearing is perfect now. Some warning signs to look for:

Newborns. Failure to startle in response to a sudden loud sound may signal trouble. This startle reflex diminishes naturally within the first few months of life, but if you don't see it in your newborn, it could signal a possible hearing loss. Infants also learn quickly to locate the source of a sound (if they hear something, they'll turn their heads in that direction) and can be calmed by certain sounds and voices, even music. If your baby cannot be calmed by his or her mother's voice by about three months of age, suspect a hearing impairment.

About three months of age. By now, babies should be able to smile when they hear their names and recognize significant voices. They may also be able to play turn-taking games: If adults say something in response to their babbling, they'll listen for a moment and then try to imitate what was said. If your baby doesn't exhibit

5 Minute Hearing Test

	Almost always	Half the time	Occasionally	Never
1. I have a problem hearing over the telephone.				
2. I have trouble following the conversation when two or more people are talking at the same time.				
3. People complain that I turn the TV volume too high.				
4. I have to strain to understand conversations.				
5. I miss hearing some common sounds like the phone or doorbell ringing.				
6. I have trouble hearing conversations in a noisy background such as a party.				
7. I get confused about where sounds come from.				
8. I misunderstand some words in a sentence and need to ask people to repeat themselves.				

9. I especially have trouble understanding the speech of women and children.			
10. I have worked in noisy environments (assembly lines, jackhammers, jet engines, etc.).			
11. Many people I talk to seem to mumble (or don't speak clearly).			
12. People get annoyed because I misunderstand what they say.			
13. I misunderstand what others are saying and make inappropriate responses.			
14. I avoid social activities because I cannot hear well and fear I'll reply improperly.			

To be answered by a family member or friend:

15. Do you think this person has a hearing loss?

Scoring

To calculate your score, give yourself 3 points for every time you checked the "Almost always" column, 2 for every "Half the time," 1 for every "Occasionally," and 0 for every "Never." If you have a blood relative who has a hearing loss, add another 3 points. Then total your points.

The American Academy of Otolaryngology—Head and Neck Surgery recommends the following:

- 0 to 5—Your hearing is fine. No action is required.
- 6 to 9—Suggest you see an ear-nose-and-throat (ENT) specialist.
- 10 and above—Strongly recommend you see an ear physician.

Credit: Reprinted with the permission of the American Academy of Otolaryngology—Head and Neck Surgery

some or all of these behaviors, it's possible he or she may be hard of hearing.

Between four and six months. Babies of this age learn to respond to changes in tone of voice and may even become distressed if, for example, adults say "No!" harshly. Once again, if your baby doesn't seem to be responding in this way, you might think of a possible hearing loss.

Seven to twelve months. At this age, children enjoy games like peekaboo and pat-a-cake. They should also know their names and certain familiar words (*mama,* for example), and their babbling, while not comprehensible to an adult, should start taking on a more purposeful sound—you'll probably be able to hear the same rhythm and intonations as in normal speech. Babies who cannot hear probably will not make these sounds.

One to two years. Most babies in this age range can point to and name familiar objects; they should also be able to follow simple commands, such as "Kiss the baby," "Roll the ball," or "Get your shoes." From about 18 months on, they should start making simple two- or three-word sentences on their own: "More milk," "Go car," and the ubiquitous "Mine, mine, mine." If a child's development of language or comprehension doesn't seem to be following these milestones, it could indicate a possible hearing loss.

The AAO-HNS has devised a checklist for people who suspect that a child may be hard of hearing. You might wish to consult it and follow their recommendations if you're truly concerned.

Don't, however, immediately assume that your child has a hearing loss simply on the basis of what you've read here. Only a doctor can make that diagnosis for sure. On the other hand, do have your child checked immediately. Today, even newborns can be fitted with hearing aids and, with their parents, placed in special programs called parent-infant training programs that teach them appropriate language and communication skills. Any large public school system should be able to provide you with more information on this program and on raising a hearing-impaired child.

Testing a baby's hearing is easy and painless and well worth the peace of mind it can bring.

FINDING THE RIGHT DOCTOR

Most hearing disorders in children or adults can be diagnosed after just a few basic tests. Some problems may require more specialized tests for precise identification, but these are rare. What's most important is to be sure that the person who examines you or your loved one is trained to identify hearing problems and treat them properly or to refer you to someone who *can* provide treatment.

HEARING SPECIALISTS

There are several types of specialists within the field of *otology,* the field of medicine concerned with the diagnosis and management of disorders of the ear and related structures. If your hearing is impaired, you'll most likely be treated by an *otolaryngologist,* a doctor who

Determining if Your Child Has a Hearing Loss

If you think that your child has a hearing loss, you might be right. The following checklist will assist in determining whether or not your child might have a hearing loss. Please read each item carefully and check *only* those factors that apply to you, your family, or your child.

RISK CRITERIA—CHECK EACH ITEM THAT APPLIES:

During Pregnancy

☐ Mother had German measles, a viral infection, or flu

☐ Mother drank alcoholic beverages

My Newborn (Birth to 28 Days of Age)

☐ Weighed less than 3.5 pounds at birth

☐ Has an unusual appearance of the face or ears

☐ Was jaundiced (yellow skin) at birth and almost had or did have an exchange blood transfusion

☐ Was in neonatal intensive care unit (NICU) for more than two days

☐ Received an antibiotic medication through a needle in a vein

☐ Had meningitis

My Family

☐ Has one or more individuals with permanent or progressive hearing loss that was present or developed early in life

My Infant (29 Days to Age Two Years)

☐ Received an antibiotic medication given through a needle in a vein

☐ Had meningitis

☐ Has a neurological disorder

☐ Had a serious injury with a fracture of the skull with or without bleeding from the ear

RESPONSE TO THE ENVIRONMENT (SPEECH AND LANGUAGE DEVELOPMENT)

Newborn (Birth to 6 Months)

☐ Does not startle, move, cry, or react in any way to unexpected loud noises

☐ Does not awaken to loud noises

☐ Does not freely imitate sound

☐ Cannot be soothed by voice alone

☐ Does not turn his/her head in the direction of my voice

Young Infant (6 Through 12 Months)

☐ Does not point to familiar persons or objects when asked

☐ Does not babble or babbling has stopped

☐ By 12 months is not understanding simple phrases such as "Wave bye bye" or "Clap hands" by listening alone

Older Infant (13 Months Through Two Years)

☐ Does not accurately turn in the direction of a soft voice on the first call

☐ Is not alert to environmental sounds

☐ Does not respond on first call

☐ Does not respond to sound or does not locate where sound is coming from

☐ Does not begin to imitate and use simple words for familiar people and things around the home

☐ Does not sound like or use speech like other children of similar age

☐ Does not listen to TV at a normal volume

☐ Does not show consistent growth in the understanding and the use of words to communicate

WHAT YOU SHOULD DO

If you have checked one or more of these factors, your child may be *at risk* for hearing loss. *At risk* simply means there is a better-than-average chance of a hearing loss.

If your child is at risk, you should take him or her for an ear examination and a hearing test. This can be done *at any age*, as early as just after birth.

If you did not check any of these factors but you suspect that your child is not hearing normally, even if your child's doctor is not concerned, have your child's hearing tested by an audiologist and, when appropriate, his or her speech evaluated by a speech and language pathologist. If no hearing loss exists, the test will not have hurt him or her. However, if your child does have a hearing loss, delayed diagnosis could affect speech and language development.

This information is provided as a public service to parents who are concerned that their child might have a hearing loss. It is not a substitute for an ear examination or a hearing test. Hearing loss can exist in children even though none of these checklist items are present.

Reprinted with the permission of the American Academy of Otolaryngology—Head and Neck Surgery.

specializes in treating disorders of the nose, throat, and neck as well as the ears. That's why these physicians often call themselves *otorhinolaryngologists* or *otolaryngologists—head and neck surgeons*. They can measure, evaluate, and treat ear disorders, prescribe medications, and project the future needs of hearing-impaired patients.

Some otolaryngologists concentrate only on treating ear disorders and hearing problems. These doctors are called *otologists*. They, too, can measure and evaluate hearing disorders and prescribe medication.

Earlier in this chapter, we mentioned the AAO-HNS, the professional organization of these specialists. To qualify for membership, the doctor must be licensed in otolaryngology and meet the training requirements set forth by the AAO-HNS. If you'd like to be checked by an otolaryngologist but don't know how to find one, the AAO-HNS makes these recommendations:

- Ask your family physician or some other doctor you trust for a referral.

- Contact your state or local medical society and ask them for a list of specialists in your area.

- To check the doctor's background and credentials, look in the current edition of the *Directory of Medical Specialists,* available in many public or medical libraries; you might also want to learn which hospital the doctor's affiliated with, in the event that you require surgery.

Another suggestion: The June 15, 1992, issue of *U.S. News & World Report* contains a list of the finest hospitals in the United States, based on the opinions of 1,000 doctors in different specialties. The hospitals named as best in otolaryngology are listed below. As you'll see, they're located across the country. If you live near one of these centers, why not call and ask if any of their staff physicians see private patients, or if the hospital itself has a clinic? If you don't live close by but are in the same state or general region of the country, perhaps someone at the hospital can refer you to a specialist closer to home. The hospitals are:

University of Iowa Hospitals and Clinics—Iowa City

Massachusetts Eye and Ear Infirmary—Boston

Johns Hopkins Hospital—Baltimore

UCLA Medical Center—Los Angeles

Mayo Clinic—Rochester, Minnesota

University of Texas (M. D. Anderson Cancer Center)—Houston

University of Michigan Medical Center—Ann Arbor

Audiologists

The person who actually tests your hearing at first may not be a medical doctor but another professional known as an *audiologist*. These individuals specialize in hearing measurement and also in the recommendation and fitting of hearing aids. When you arrive for your initial hearing tests, it'll probably be the audiologist who performs these tests, even if it's in the doctor's office. Audiologists consider themselves communication specialists because they offer support and counseling to help people deal with hearing disabilities. Some audiologists even teach lipreading and other kinds of hearing and speech training.

Minimal training for an audiologist includes a master's degree plus at least one year of training under the aegis of a more experienced audiologist. Many audiologists go on to earn a Ph.D. and participate in teaching and research. A word of warning: Some people who fit and sell hearing aids may call themselves "audiologists" but are really not. Only someone who's gone through the training described above is entitled to call himself or herself an audiologist. If you have any reason to doubt someone's credentials, ask the individual what degrees he or she has and where he or she was trained. Remember, an audiologist must have at least a master's degree in a field such as audiology or hearing and speech rehabilitation.

HEARING TESTS

Most people undergo a standard series of tests initially. Then, depending on the results of these tests, your doctor or audiologist may recommend a more specialized evaluation to determine exactly what your problem is and how it should be treated.

Standard Tests

Medical and Personal History. The information gleaned from your work, family, and medical history is indispensable to a correct diagnosis. For example, if you tell the doctor you've been a construction worker for 20 years, and your hearing loss is mostly in the range of

3,000 to 6,000 Hz (these are considered fairly high frequencies), he'll most likely conclude you've got noise-induced hearing loss. If you're a woman who first noticed a hearing loss shortly after becoming pregnant or giving birth, and tests indicate your loss is mostly in the lower frequencies, chances are the doctor will diagnose a condition known as *otosclerosis,* described below.

It's essential that you tell the doctor about all the medications you're taking. Volunteer the information in the unlikely event that he doesn't ask about it. Among the drugs known to affect hearing are:

• Aspirin

• Quinine

• Sulfa drugs

• Antihistamines

• Antibiotics: dihydrostreptomycin, kanamycin, streptomycin, neomycin, and vancomycin

Pure-Tone Hearing Test.   This test, usually one of the first you'll undergo, measures your ability to hear certain frequencies by presenting you with sounds at the lowest volume you can hear. Each sound is a *pure tone,* which is a tone composed of only one frequency (in the real world, most sounds consist of several frequencies). You'll be shown into a soundproof room and given a pair of headphones to put on—actually, this will be the case with most of the tests discussed here. Through the headphones, you'll hear sounds of differing frequency and volume, presented first to one ear, then the other. This will be done by the audiologist, who will probably be sitting in the room with you or in an adjoining room equipped with a window through which he or she can see you. You'll be instructed to indicate when you can hear each sound— probably by raising your hand. By measuring the decibel level, or volume, at which you can hear each frequency, the audiologist can determine your hearing threshold for each frequency. From this information, he or she creates a graph, called an *audiogram,* depicting your threshold for each frequency you've heard. The audiogram gives doctors and audiologists an easy way to determine quickly the degree of your hearing impairment, if any, and which frequencies are particularly affected. This test takes approximately 20 to 30 minutes.

Discomfort Level. If the audiologist wants to check your sensitivity to loudness, he or she will raise the volume on some or all of the pure tones and have you indicate when it becomes uncomfortably loud. In a different version of the test, he or she may have you listen to a recording of someone speaking, again through the earphones, and have you indicate your discomfort level to speech at differing volumes.

Speech Hearing or Discrimination Test. In this test, you'll hear a series of words through earphones or through a loudspeaker. You'll hear one set of words at differing volume levels, then another at a volume that's comfortable for you. To indicate your ability to understand each word, you'll be asked to repeat it. Thus, the audiologist sees if you can discriminate between the words *cat* and *cap,* or *fame* and *same,* for example, both at a normal conversational level and when the volume is raised. This test usually takes about 15 to 20 minutes.

With these basic tests and information, your doctor and audiologist can determine a lot about the nature of your hearing loss: the frequencies and volume levels affected and your ability to understand speech.

On the other hand, not all problems are diagnosed so easily. If the doctor or audiologist needs more information to determine exactly what's causing your hearing loss, he or she may perform more-specialized tests, such as the following.

Bone Conduction Tests. The basic tests described above measure the ability to hear through air conduction. If these tests suggest that your hearing is abnormal, your bone conduction hearing may also be evaluated. For this test, a special device, which vibrates at certain frequencies, will be placed on the mastoid bone behind the ear, and you'll be asked to report what, if anything, you hear. This test involves only the inner ear; the outer and middle ears are bypassed. Better hearing on the bone conduction test than through the earphones tells the doctor that you have a conductive hearing impairment—that the outer or middle ears are affected but not the inner ear.

Impedance and Acoustic Reflex Tests.   If the problem does indeed seem to originate in the middle ear, you may undergo a series of tests known as *impedance audiometry*, which further evaluates the function of middle ear structures including the eustachian tube and middle ear muscles, as well as middle ear pressure and the acoustic nerve. For impedance audiometry, the audiologist inserts a small measuring device (it looks like an earplug) into your ear canal. This delivers a low-pitched humming sound, along with occasional minute changes in pressure that are designed to simulate the pressure variations you'd feel if you were changing altitude, as in an airplane. The audiologist will be able to measure your response to these changes automatically; you won't have to do a thing. The test lasts about 15 to 25 minutes.

Balance Tests (Electronystagmography). The mechanism responsible for helping you maintain normal balance is located in the middle ear. Often, damage to inner ear structures may affect the balance apparatus. Or you may simply complain of feeling dizzy or be especially prone to seasickness. In these cases, the doctor will perform a test called *electronystagmography,* or *ENG.*

For ENG, some electrodes will be taped to your face, and you'll be asked to lie down. The audiologist or technician will squirt cool water into one ear for thirty seconds, followed by warm water; then the process will be repeated on the other ear. After each irrigation, he or she will observe your eye movements, which reflect the action of the balance mechanism and which will be recorded automatically by the facial electrodes. The test is completely painless, although some people experience a little discomfort during irrigation. The test takes about an hour.

There's now a variation on the standard ENG test, called *infrared* or *video ENG.* You don't need to lie down for this test, and only cold water will be irrigated through the ears to stimulate the balance mechanism. Before the test, you'll don special goggles that are hooked up to a video camera, which records your eye movements on a television screen as the water is placed in your ears. Like the standard ENG, video ENG lasts about one hour.

Because these tests measure balance, it's wise to avoid

medications that prevent or relieve dizziness or seasickness for at least 48 hours before the test and would include products such as over-the-counter seasickness patches or seasickness remedies such as Bonine or Dramamine. In addition, you'll probably be instructed to forgo some prescription tranquilizers or sedatives. It's also a good idea to abstain from alcohol for at least 24 hours before an ENG.

Electrocochleography. If the basic tests indicate you have a problem in the inner ear, *electrocochleography* may help determine the exact location of the inner ear defect. After administering a local anesthetic, the doctor will insert a tiny electrode through your eardrum, then present you with certain sounds to listen to. The electrode registers the response of your inner ear and hearing nerve to these sound stimuli. The information is then fed into a computer, which ultimately helps the doctor determine the exact nature of the inner ear disturbance. The test can be done in the doctor's office and lasts an hour to an hour and a half.

Auditory Brain Stem Response Audiometry. This test may also be performed if the doctor suspects an inner ear defect. As the name implies, it can identify problems affecting the brain stem, as well as the inner ear. To conduct the test, small disks (electrodes) will be placed around your ear and scalp, and you'll listen to a series of sounds. The electrodes record your brain's response to those sounds and feed the information to a computer. One of the advantages of this test is that because it requires no response from the person being tested, it can be performed on people who may be unable to indicate their hearing loss in any other way, such as babies.

In most cases, the tests discussed here should provide all the information a doctor needs to diagnose your hearing loss. If they don't, there are other, more sophisticated tests available, most of which measure nerve and brain function in more detail. Such tests may not be available to community doctors or hospitals; so in rare cases, patients must travel to major hearing clinics in big cities to have these tests performed. Fortunately, the vast majority of hearing disorders present straightforward diagnostic challenges.

COMMON DIAGNOSES

In Chapter Two, you saw how conductive, sensorineural, and mixed hearing impairments resulted from dysfunction in the outer, middle, or inner ears, and you learned how environmental agents such as noise often damage the ear. Taken together, these factors produce a few very common hearing disorders, one of which your doctor will most likely diagnose after he or she knows the results of your tests. Among the most common hearing problems are:

Presbycusis

Presbycusis is the medical term for the sensorineural hearing loss that comes with age. In 1982, some 6 million American adults aged 65 or more were thought to have presbycusis. By the year 2000, that number may be as high as 8 million. Some experts claim that presbycusis may occur in any adult who lives long enough, but that may not be true, as we'll discuss below.

In most people—or most Americans anyway—the ability to hear starts to diminish measurably as early as age 20, especially in men (the severity of the loss is also greater in men). Hearing in the higher-frequency ranges goes first. In fact, babies often can hear extremely high-pitched sounds that a 20-year-old can't detect. Usually, hearing weakens in both ears simultaneously. Along with loss of high-frequency hearing, disproportionate sensitivity to loud sounds is also characteristic of presbycusis.

Presbycusis may begin around age 20, but it usually doesn't become noticeable until age 50 or so, although some people may notice a hearing loss in their midforties. As many as 25 percent of people in their sixties and seventies may have a noticeable hearing deficit.

Presbycusis is thought to result from the deterioration of hair cells in the cochlea that comes with age. As the hair cells wither away, they no longer can respond to sound properly. The cells that conduct high-frequency sounds deteriorate first, which is why high-frequency hearing is the first to be impaired. This damage may be caused or compounded by excessive noise, which also damages hair cells and causes hearing loss in the higher frequencies.

Other medical problems common in older people may contribute to the hearing loss seen with presbycusis. Heart disease or high blood pressure may diminish the blood supply to ear structures; this, in turn, may cause stiffening of the ossicles and/or thickening and stiffening of the eardrum, either of which may impair sound con-

duction through the ear. The resulting hearing impairment adds to the sensorineural impairment caused by
presbycusis.

Age-related hearing loss is so common in Western society that many people just assume it's an inevitable part of
aging. However, this is not necessarily the case. The fact
is, there are parts of the world in which men and women
retain perfect hearing until well into old age; usually, they
live relatively stress-free lives in quiet surroundings. Many
experts now believe that a number of factors contribute to
the development of presbycusis: the constant level of
noise to which we're exposed; conditions such as heart
disease and high blood pressure, which result from a poor
diet and a sedentary life-style; stress; and possibly heredity
as well. So the *bad* news about presbycusis is that so many
aspects of our lives seem to promote its development; but
the *good* news is that poor hearing needn't be an ines-
capable part of aging. On the other hand, if you *do* have
presbycusis, don't blame yourself. You may have inherited
a tendency for it, and there is still much about it that isn't
known for sure.

Otosclerosis

Otosclerosis is an inherited condition in which soft,
spongy bone grows around the stirrup and oval window,
causing the stirrup to become fixed in place and impeding
the conduction of sound to the inner ear. Sometimes,
otosclerosis may spread to the inner ear, adding a sensorineural component to the hearing loss.

Interestingly, many people with no apparent hearing
loss later turn out to have the physiological signs of oto-

sclerosis. Therefore, even though the condition is hereditary, it's possible to find hearing loss due to otosclerosis
in someone with no known family history of the disease.
That's because some people seem to have the spongy
growth *without* the hearing loss, while a relative may exhibit both traits. So the condition may go undetected in a
family until one or more members start to lose their hearing.

In the United States, 66 percent of the people with otosclerosis are white women. It's rare in blacks and most
people of Asian descent but is quite common in India.
Hearing loss first starts to appear in the late teens or early
twenties, but occasionally it may occur in people older or
younger. Often, otosclerosis worsens or first begins when
a woman becomes pregnant. Cynthia, mentioned at the
beginning of this chapter, had otosclerosis.

Once otosclerosis develops, its course is chronic and
progressive. Hearing impairment may be quite rapid in
some people; usually, it starts as a mild loss in volume
and continues until the individual has lost 40 to 50 db
worth of hearing, then it levels off. Most people with otosclerosis can benefit from hearing aids or surgery. Surgery for otosclerosis is a delicate operation that requires a
lot of practice, but it is commonly performed by ear specialists. During the operation, the doctor removes the
spongy bone that's grown in the middle ear and replaces
it with a prosthesis. The outcome of the surgery is usually
good in over 90 percent of patients: As one woman put it,
"I was completely deaf before the operation, but as soon
as I woke up, I could hear again!"

Ménière's Disease

Named for the French physician Prosper Ménière, who first diagnosed the condition in 1861, Ménière's disease is a form of nerve deafness caused by the accumulation of fluid in the inner ear. Its major symptoms include episodes of fluctuating hearing loss, ringing in the ears, dizziness, a sensation of fullness in the ears, nausea, and ear pain. Most of these symptoms are due to increased pressure in the inner ear fluid. The first symptoms of Ménière's disease usually appear between the ages of 35 and 55, most often in women. Usually, the ability to hear low-pitched sounds deteriorates first, followed by loss of hearing in the higher frequencies. Episodes of Ménière's disease are usually confined to one ear, and typically the hearing gets worse with each bout.

Ménière's disease is still something of a mystery because no one knows what causes it; the symptoms may come and go without explanation. An episode may be preceded by tinnitus or a feeling of fullness in the ear, or it may occur without warning. The dizziness or vertigo associated with Ménière's disease may last from a few minutes to as long as several hours; people with this condition describe feelings of violent spinning, whirling, falling, and nausea and vomiting. Usually, the first attack is the worst; subsequent episodes are shorter and milder and may not occur until years after the initial episode.

People with Ménière's disease often report episodes occurring in close conjunction with periods of grief, pressure, or frustration in their lives. And of course, the symptoms themselves can produce a lot of stress. Some people believe that Ménière's disease may be caused by allergies, although this theory is controversial. According to reports dating back to the 1920s, symptoms of Ménière's disease appeared in some people following exposure to items they were allergic to, like certain foods or airborne allergens (dust, pollen). As yet, this theory hasn't been put to any rigorous tests, but if you've been diagnosed with Ménière's disease and you have allergies, try keeping track of your exposure to the allergens and see if there's any association with the symptoms of Ménière's disease. Include the type of allergen, the time of day, intensity of the exposure, and length of time between exposure to the allergens and the development of Ménière's disease symptoms. Try avoiding the allergen if you can and see if that decreases the frequency or intensity of your symptoms. Consistency in the worsening of symptoms following exposure to a particular substance is an especially important tip-off to a possible relationship between Ménière's disease and any allergies you might have.

Because no one knows what causes Ménière's disease, it can't be treated directly. Instead, therapy is aimed at relieving the symptoms when they occur. This seems to help about 80 percent of the patients treated. You may be instructed to avoid caffeine, alcohol, and cigarettes; to follow a low-salt diet; and to avoid noise and stress as much as possible. These precautions have been found to diminish the frequency of attacks in many people. People in whom medical treatment proves inadequate may undergo surgery, the type of operation depending on the degree of vertigo or hearing loss. First, the surgeon might insert a tube in a membrane of the inner ear so that some of the accumulated fluid can drain away and be absorbed by the surrounding tissue. This procedure seems to help about 75 percent of those on whom it's performed.

However, if that doesn't work, and if the patient's vertigo is really severe, the doctor may attempt a more drastic procedure: cutting the portion of the eighth nerve associated with balance. Unfortunately, some people who undergo this operation often feel very dizzy afterward for periods ranging from a few days to as long as a few months, although it tapers off gradually. The brighter side is that the episodes of vertigo cease; and many sufferers of Ménière's disease derive great comfort from knowing that they've endured their last episode of this troubling disorder. Because any operation has risks, this step should be reserved only for those people whose vertigo is intense and who cannot be helped in any other way. Fortunately, their numbers are relatively few, and the surgery's success rate is high: over 90 percent.

Surgery often relieves the severe dizziness afflicting people with Ménière's disease, but there's no guarantee that it will restore hearing: Some people improve; others actually get worse. However, many patients choose an operation anyway to escape the incapacitating dizziness they may experience.

All in all, diagnosing a hearing problem is not difficult. You may wonder, however, how you developed such a problem in the first place. Often, an individual has little, if any, control over the things that affect hearing—heredity or viruses, for example. In other cases, you might be able to prevent hearing damage to some degree, as with noise-related injury. Chapter Four describes in more detail some of the most significant causes of hearing loss: noise, infections, injuries, and other problems. It also includes some suggestions on how to protect your hearing as best you can. From there, you'll learn in the following chapters how to cope with a hearing loss, be it yours or that of a loved one, and how to go on with an active, fulfilling, independent—in other words, normal—life.

PREVENTING HEARING LOSS

Now you know something about the normal hearing process and what can go wrong. Is there anything you can do to protect your ears and your hearing? Sometimes there is. To learn more about preventing hearing loss, let's first take a closer look at some of the major causes of hearing loss that were introduced in earlier chapters. Then we'll look at ways you can preserve your hearing.

OUR NOISY WORLD

Of the roughly 28 million Americans with hearing loss, some 10 million of those people owe their impairment at least in part to noise. It is by far the most significant single cause of hearing loss in the United States and probably in most of Western society.

Noise injury occurs from all sorts of sounds we hear every day—on and off the job, in urban and rural areas, day in and day out. Perhaps you've told your kids they're going to ruin their hearing listening to that loud music they seem to adore. But did you know that motors on speedboats, motorcycles, and even lawn mowers may be just as harmful? In addition, you might warn your kids that too much time playing pinball or video games may also damage their hearing. And if their friends seem to call nonstop, now you've got the perfect way to discourage them: The ring on some cordless phones is apparently loud enough and strident enough to harm the ears.

It seems that noise is getting harder and harder to escape in our society. Even spacecraft are noisy: Astronauts have reported problems sleeping, concentrating, and relaxing while in flight, and many of them show signs of temporary hearing loss when they return to earth. Scientists recently determined that noise levels aboard the space shuttle *Columbia,* which orbited the earth in June 1991, were a constant 70 db—comparable with the noise of a busy freeway and enough to cause a small but significant hearing loss in the crew.

These findings support something doctors have known for years: Continual exposure to moderately loud noise is the cause of the most insidious, and probably the most common, form of hearing loss associated with noise.

Noise-Induced Hearing Loss

Ear damage from noise is so ubiquitous in today's world that doctors have given it a name: *noise-induced hearing loss,* or *NIHL.* Usually, NIHL occurs in both ears, but it doesn't have to. One ear may suffer more damage than the other if, for example, you've been exposed to more noise on one side. For instance, people who regularly fire rifles experience more NIHL in the ear on the side on which they hold the rifle.

How does noise damage our hearing? Doctors don't have all the answers yet, but it does seem clear that one way is through damage to the hair cells in the cochlea. There's some evidence that excessive noise causes temporary changes in certain portions of the hair cells, which in turn diminish hearing sensitivity—a *temporary threshold shift,* or *TTS.* Experimental animals exposed repeatedly to sounds that cause TTS eventually sustain permanent hearing loss.

The pitch, or frequency, of the sound also makes a difference. If you're exposed for a moderate period of time to a potentially hazardous, high-frequency sound, any damage that occurs will probably be confined to that region of the cochlea that detects high-frequency sound. But if you spend the same amount of time listening to potentially hazardous *low*-frequency noise, you'll damage hair cells in both the high- and low-frequency areas of the cochlea —and hair cells are *not* replaceable. The pattern of damage will also reflect factors such as the acoustic properties of the ear canal, the condition of the middle ear, and the mechanical characteristics of the organ of Corti and other components of the inner ear. Obviously, continued exposure to hazardous sound will damage more and more hair cells.

TTS often occurs after a moderate period of sound exposure, but if that episode is followed by some relative peace and quiet, your hearing threshold should return to normal. If the noise exposure continues regularly, it may cause a *permanent threshold shift,* or *PTS.* The more noise, the more serious the PTS will be, and the broader range of frequencies it will encompass. As noise exposure persists, NIHL will increase rapidly, especially in the early years of its development. Finally, after many years of exposure, NIHL usually levels off in the high frequencies, although it may continue to worsen at lower frequencies. Unfortunately, the magnitude of TTS can't be used to predict the magnitude of PTS or the ultimate degree of NIHL.

Which Sounds Are Worst?

Hearing loss can't be traced only to one kind of sound. To determine if a particular sound will damage someone's hearing, doctors must know something about the duration of that person's exposure to the sound: how many minutes or hours in a typical day, and how many months or years. This holds for all kinds of sounds, such as rock music, snowmobiles, and chain saws. So before you warn your kids that they're ruining their hearing, try to have some idea of how *often* they're actually listening to their music and for *how long*. Most sounds that cause permanent threshold shifts in hearing do so after long exposure: eight hours a day, five days a week, for ten or more years. There are indeed some noises that may damage hearing after a single exposure (one example might be a shotgun blast in combat), but it's hard to predict what these are because everyone's susceptibility is different.

According to most experts, however, *occupation* is the most common cause of NIHL. The highest-risk jobs include:

Fire fighting

Police work

Military service

Construction and factory work

Music industry

Farming

Driving a truck

If you work in any of these areas, it's probably a good idea to have regular hearing tests.

As for nonoccupational sounds, those that seem to be hardest on the ears include:

Loud music

Recreational vehicles

Airplanes

Lawn mowers

Woodworking tools

Chain saws

Some household appliances like the cordless phones mentioned earlier

Most doctors agree that sounds below 75 db of volume probably won't cause permanent hearing loss even at high frequencies. With louder noises, however, the amount of hearing loss will be related to the sound level. This is especially apparent with sound louder than 85 db; at that level, prolonged exposure will almost certainly cause some hearing loss after many years.

At lower noise levels, some experiments have demonstrated that a volume of 60 to 65 db—about the volume of a normal conversation—is enough to annoy about 9 percent of the people asked but not loud enough to cause NIHL.

How Do I Know if a Sound Is Hazardous?

If you live or work in a noisy environment, learn some of the tip-offs of a potentially hazardous sound. Your hearing may be in jeopardy:

- If the sound is appreciably louder than conversational level and is of sufficiently long duration.

- If the sound makes it difficult to communicate, if you experience tinnitus after hearing the sound, or if other sounds seem muffled after you leave the environment in which you're exposed to the sound in question.

Also, remember that no two people will respond in exactly the same way to a sound. Just because your coworkers don't seem to be bothered by a particular sound—and you are—doesn't mean you're a hypochondriac. Similarly, the noise that you hardly pay attention to may be driving the person next to you crazy. In fact, there may be as much as a 35- to 50-db difference in the sounds that cause temporary or permanent threshold shifts in different people. So if the noise in your environment bothers *you,* have your ears checked and take the appropriate measures to protect your hearing (some suggestions are given later in this chapter).

No one knows exactly why these differences exist, but it probably has something to do with the amount of total wear and tear on each person's ears, combined with in-born differences in anatomy and physiology. Gender seems to play a role: Between the ages of 10 and 20, men's hearing becomes measurably worse than women's, a difference that continues into old age. This probably has less to do with any inborn differences than with the fact that men more frequently choose jobs and leisure activities in which they're more likely to be exposed to excessive noise.

Consequences of Noise-Induced Hearing Loss

People with NIHL usually lose high-frequency hearing first. Perhaps one of the most insidious consequences of this process is the loss of the ability to understand speech. With hearing loss in the higher-frequency ranges, important speech information becomes inaudible or incomprehensible. For example, consonants are high-frequency sounds. Someone who can't distinguish between *p, t,* or *b* sounds won't be able to tell the words *cap, cat,* and *cab* apart. Other interfering sounds—such as background noise, competing voices, or room reverberations—may reduce hearing ability even further. Tinnitus, which is for many people another symptom of NIHL, makes the situation even worse. Fortunately, there are ways to compensate for most of these problems, as you'll see in Chapter Six.

What can be done to prevent, or at least diminish, the problem of noise-induced hearing loss, at least in the workplace? A panel recently convened by the National Institutes of Health made these recommendations:

- Managers should have sound surveys performed to assess the degree of hazardous noise exposure.

- People in high-risk jobs should be shown ways they can minimize hearing loss at work; they should also be provided with equipment to protect hearing, such as earplugs, earmuffs, and canal caps that fit directly into the ear canal. Currently, standards set by the Occupational Safety and Health Administration (OSHA) require workers exposed to noise louder than 85 db more than eight hours a day to have hearing protection.

- In addition, workers in high-risk environments should receive regular hearing tests so that any loss can be detected early.

- Government regulations that currently apply to most noisy industries should be revised to encompass *all* industries and all employees, strengthened in certain areas, and strictly enforced, with more inspections and more severe penalties for violations.

- Organization and staff training should be improved in hearing-protection programs that already exist.

Noise pollution in the United States isn't just an individual health problem; it may affect nothing less than our ability to compete in the world marketplace. At a recent meeting of the American Acoustical Society (an organization of physicists, audiologists, engineers, architects, and specialists in other fields, all concerned with acoustical problems), a German scientist noted that Europe is now developing a uniform set of environmental standards, including some involving noise, that will ultimately affect some 380 million people. He warned that unless American companies comply with these standards, American competitiveness in Europe will suffer.

OTITIS MEDIA

Otitis media is another common cause of hearing loss and probably is the most common single cause of conductive hearing impairment. Fortunately, the hearing loss associated with it is often temporary, but if the infection isn't detected and treated in time, permanent damage may result. So prompt recognition and care are the keys to preventing permanent hearing loss induced by otitis media.

Otitis Media in Children

As every parent knows, these infections are especially prevalent in children; according to some estimates, up to two thirds of all American toddlers suffer at least one bout of otitis media before they start school. Children seem to be particular targets of middle ear infection because their middle ear structure has not yet matured: A child's eustachian tube is shorter and more horizontal in position than that of an adult. These qualities make it easier for viruses and other "bugs" that cause colds and upper respiratory tract infections to enter the eustachian tube and spread to the middle ear. Simultaneously, mucus or pus can accumulate in the middle ear and fail to drain away. Thus, the middle ear becomes inflamed, swollen, painful, and filled with fluid—the classic symptoms of otitis media. Hearing may seem muffled, or voices may carry an echo.

Complications

As stated above, any associated hearing loss is usually temporary but may become permanent if the infection isn't treated quickly or aggressively enough. Otitis media is a good example of a condition that's simple to treat in its early stages but that can turn serious, even life-threatening, if ignored for too long. The infection may spread to the mastoid bone, which houses the ear, leading to a condition called *mastoiditis*, which is sometimes fatal. Pain that occurs behind the ear, especially if it's in conjunction with otitis media, is a tip-off to possible mastoiditis. Usually, doctors hospitalize people with this condition and administer intravenous antibiotics. They may also perform minor surgery to drain the middle ear. More serious cases of mastoiditis may require more extensive surgery, as described in Chapter Six.

Serous Otitis Media

Most uncomplicated cases of otitis media respond to antibiotics and leave no permanent damage. However, prompt treatment is essential, mainly to avoid the risk of mastoiditis but also to prevent the buildup of fluid behind the eardrum. Sometimes the eardrum bursts from the pressure; again, fast treatment can help the eardrum heal without any loss of hearing. Without this, permanent hearing loss may occur. Possible symptoms of this kind of infection, called *serous* or *perforated otitis media,* are a discharge and crusting around the outer ear, from fluid leaking out from the perforated eardrum. Some patients feel nothing at all when the eardrum bursts; others report a jolt of intense ear pain that then diminishes, possibly followed by blood or mucus draining from the ear. Fortunately, once the eardrum has ruptured and drained, most cases of serous otitis media resolve on their own.

Treatment for serous otitis media usually consists of a two-week course of antibiotics, mostly to decrease the risk of mastoiditis or meningitis. Some doctors also prescribe ear drops. Until the eardrum is healed and the infection completely gone, patients are usually warned not to get their ears wet, because that may slow down the healing process. Sometimes, to let the fluid drain away completely, the doctor may make a small incision in the eardrum, which then heals spontaneously. However, if the fluid buildup persists, he or she may insert a small drainage tube in the eardrum. This is painless and can safely stay in place for as long as a year. There is a slight risk that the tube may become dislodged, or that the body may reject it, but for the most part, the eardrum heals over eventually and the tube falls harmlessly out of the ear.

Chronic Otitis Media

Some children are prone to a condition called *chronic otitis media* in which they suffer repeated bouts of infection, as many as five to six episodes each year. These episodes sometimes take the form of serous otitis media, because fluid accumulation may cause the eardrum to burst. Children with chronic otitis media bear careful watching because the recurrent infections may cause lasting ear damage. No one knows why some children are more susceptible than others to these persistent infections, but one theory holds that after the body fights off the initial infection, some residual germs remain, presenting the immune system with a constant, low level of stimulation. This, in turn, may be what leads to the fluid buildup in the ear.

In children, numerous bouts of infection may lead to permanent hearing loss. The auditory system needs the regular stimulus of sound to develop properly. Periodic episodes of hearing loss, even if they're only temporary, may deprive maturing ear structures of the sound they need, ultimately causing lasting hearing impairment and interfering with the child's development of speech and language skills. Since there's often little or no pain accompanying chronic otitis media, the best danger signal is probably a decline in your child's hearing in conjunction with a cold, the flu, or an allergy attack.

OTHER EAR INFECTIONS

Otitis Externa

On the subject of otitis (this is really just a general term meaning "ear infection"), we should mention another common condition: otitis externa, or external ear infection, more popularly known as *swimmer's ear*. Water trapped in the ear canal can promote the growth of fungus or bacteria, which then infect the canal and lead to itching, swelling, and a blocked feeling in the ear. Pain, especially when you move the outer ear, may occur in more advanced cases. Fortunately, otitis externa seldom damages hearing, except for the temporary muffled sensation many people encounter when the ear canal is swollen. Other than swimming, the causes of otitis externa include (1) frequent and vigorous use of cotton swabs to clean the ears and (2) excessive scratching of itchy ears.

Otitis externa usually isn't serious, but it does require a doctor's care to resolve completely. He or she will usually prescribe a course of antibiotic ear drops for seven to ten days and warn you not to get your ears wet.

Labyrinthitis

Labyrinthitis is a viral infection of the cochlea. People with labyrinthitis develop sensorineural hearing loss plus a severe form of vertigo that makes them feel as if the room is constantly spinning. To relieve the symptoms of vertigo, your doctor may prescribe medicine that suppresses the activity of the vestibular apparatus, or a mild tranquilizer. Fortunately, the infection usually resolves on its own, and the symptoms diminish along with it.

FOREIGN OBJECTS

Foreign objects lodged in the ear are another common cause for conductive hearing loss. If you or someone you know experiences a sudden hearing loss accompanied by pain and discharge from the ear, there's a good chance it's due to something stuck in the ear. *Don't attempt to re-*

move it yourself—you may do more damage. See a doctor
as soon as possible and let him or her take it out.

As you might have guessed, this problem occurs most
commonly in children. The best way to prevent it is to
teach your child *never* to put anything in his or her ears.
A quick glance into each ear at bathtime, at bedtime, or
after your child has come in from playing might also add
to your peace of mind.

EARDRUM INJURIES

Eardrum injuries, too, occur more often than you might
realize. Many things may damage an eardrum:

- *A sharp blow to the ear.* The eardrum usually heals
  normally following such trauma, but occasionally
  permanent hearing loss does result.

- *Poking something into the ear.* That's one reason
  why you should let a doctor remove any foreign
  objects; it's also the reason why you shouldn't try
  cleaning your ears with cotton swabs, fingers, or
  anything else.

- *Blast injuries.* These are injuries that might occur
  from exposure to explosions or gunfire during combat
  or from close proximity to fireworks.

- *Any accident that fractures the bony ring in the skull
  to which the eardrum is attached.* One tip-off that
  the eardrum may have been injured is bleeding from
  the ear. Also, any accident that damages the bones of
  the middle ear may also harm the eardrum.

- *Severe middle ear infection.* Any severe middle ear infection that goes untreated for too long may eventually progress to the eardrum and damage it.

In general, muffled hearing is one tip-off to the fact that the eardrum may be affected. As mentioned earlier, an injured eardrum often heals on its own; if it doesn't, doctors can repair it with surgery, and they can also realign middle ear bones that might be damaged.

EAR CARE

Hearing loss results from many factors over which we normally have little or no control, such as accidents, noise on the job, or certain illnesses. However, there are some measures you can take to minimize your chances of contracting some ear infections, to detect potential hearing problems early enough to be treated, and to protect against the ravages of noise.

Basic Ear Care

Have your family doctor check your ears once a year for wax buildup or other problems. Some experts also recommend that adults have a thorough hearing examination once, including the basic tests mentioned in Chapter Three, and then go for reexaminations at three to five-year intervals (unless, of course, you experience hearing loss or balance problems).

As far as ear hygiene is concerned, washing the outer structure using a washcloth or tissue is usually sufficient.

Once again, remember that anything small enough to be inserted into the ear canal can inadvertently damage the eardrum; so the *best* way to avoid eardrum injury is to avoid putting anything in your ear. If your ears feel blocked from too much wax or anything else, see a doctor about removal. Avoid ear infections by swimming only in pools that have been adequately treated with chlorine. Do not swim in bodies of water known to be contaminated or polluted. And, of course, if you contract a cold or other respiratory tract infection, treat it promptly to minimize its chances of spreading to the middle ear. Whenever possible, keep your child away from other children with middle ear infections.

Noise Protection

The employers of people who work in noisy environments should provide protective devices for the ears, as described earlier. If your employer doesn't, discuss the problem with your immediate superior, shop steward, or personnel manager. Employers who run small, informal businesses may agree to reimburse you for a good pair of earplugs or earmuffs, which you can buy from an audiologist, a gun store, or even some large sporting goods stores. The most effective of these devices should provide about 30 db worth of protection; if the noise is especially loud, you may find you need the earplugs *and* earmuffs.

As for extracurricular activities, the same precautions apply. If you go to a lot of rock concerts or spend your spare time at a shooting range, some form of hearing protection is advisable. It probably isn't realistic to expect someone to wear earmuffs at a rock concert, but earplugs can be unobtrusive and are better than nothing. (And, of course, it's wise not to get too close to the stage and speakers.) In general, if you find that you experience the symptoms associated with noise damage described above, such as tinnitus or temporary hearing loss, after engaging in a particular activity on or off the job, it's probably a good idea for you to use some hearing protection—and have your hearing checked!

As you can see, doctors know quite a bit about the causes of hearing loss and how to diagnose them. And as described in this chapter and the one before it, most hearing-impaired people have fairly common, easily recognized conditions.

But what then? Does it mean you are condemned to live in a silent world—or at least a terribly quiet one? Does it mean you'll have to limit your activities or never be quite sure of what's being said? Will you have to depend on others to do things for you? In other words, are you now handicapped?

The answer is, in the great majority of cases, emphatically no. To be sure, you'll have to make some changes in your life-style, and you may have to adjust to certain things—music may never sound the same as it once did, for example. And just as certainly, there are people who are so profoundly deaf that they must rely on special methods of communication, such as sign language. But even those people can live independently, have satisfying social and work lives, and in general manage their affairs quite well. In fact, hearing-impaired people can do just about anything that anyone else can do—there are even dance troupes composed entirely of deaf people.

These people have seen to it that their lives go on by

taking advantage of the wonderful array of assistance that's available to the hearing impaired. You'll learn more about that in Chapters Six and Seven: assistive devices, hearing aids, cochlear implants, special training, support groups—even hearing-ear dogs. But to be truly ready to get on with your life, you've first got to acknowledge the fact that you've got a hearing impairment. In Chapter Five, you'll learn how you or a loved one can cope with the emotional toll of a hearing loss—the essential ingredient for a normal life.

FIVE

COPING WITH HEARING LOSS

Charlie's Story

Charlie was ecstatic—after 40 years with his company, in a job he loved, he retired in style. His colleagues threw him a great party, and best of all, he had a substantial pension and generous health benefits.

But Rita, Charlie's wife of 30 years, was not so thrilled. What Charlie had thought of as loving his job, Rita defined as workaholism. While he was putting in long hours and short vacations, she had to do things alone or with friends and had to grope for answers to the persistent questions, "Where's Charlie? Why doesn't he ever come with you?" Even when he took time off, Charlie was perfectly content to stay home and watch television and perhaps order in a pizza. Rita loved her husband—as he loved her—but she had years ago given up her dream of spending an affluent retirement traveling, perhaps moving to a warmer climate, and doing all the things she'd promised herself they'd do when Charlie had the time.

The truth was, she resented Charlie's unwillingness to share her interests.

Charlie had been retired about six months when things began to change. Despite their differences, he and Rita had gotten along as well as any two people who'd been married for so long. But now it seemed to him that she'd developed a lisp. And she began mumbling a lot. He remembered one night when she tried to tell him something while they were watching television. "Darned if I could hear a thing she said," he later told his daughter Anne. "Your mother must be getting old." Rita, in turn, said on a separate occasion, "I don't think your father's adjusting well to his retirement. Sometimes he just stares off into space, even after I say something to him. And then when I say he's not listening to me, he bites my head off! He's getting too cranky—I think he misses work."

Anne had suspected for several years that her father had a hearing problem. Neither of her parents ever brought it up (nor did she), but Anne did find it annoying sometimes to say something to her father and have him sit there without responding, as if she weren't in the room, or to repeat something to him three or four times —usually shouting the last repetition—and then have him tell her to speak more clearly. Anne tolerated these problems because she didn't see her parents that often anymore and didn't want things to be unpleasant when they were together. But several months after Charlie's retirement, her patience gave way. She'd been under a lot of stress in her own life (her husband's job was in jeopardy, and they had run up more debt than was wise), and she looked forward just to a few days away from all of that. Nevertheless, one evening, as she was trying to tell *her father about her fears, he interrupted her several times to ask, "What? Whadja say? I can't hear you. . . . Why don't you speak more clearly?" Finally, after the fourth such interruption, she could stand it no longer. "Damn it, Dad!" she screamed. "Why don't you get a hearing aid?" And then she left the room.*

DENIAL OF HEARING LOSS

Hearing loss is frightening because it affects our ability to interact with the world around us. Loss of vision is tragic, but if their hearing is unaffected, people who are completely blind still can understand what's said to them, respond appropriately, and communicate their own thoughts clearly. When individuals don't respond to something that's been said, or respond with an answer that doesn't make sense, many people may conclude that their intellect is impaired as well as their hearing. That's especially true if the hearing-impaired person is starting to get along in years. And perhaps because hearing loss is so common in elderly people in our society, many of us associate hearing loss with aging.

Maybe that's why it can be so hard to acknowledge it when we find ourselves becoming a little hard of hearing. Perhaps we want to hold off the ravages of old age as long as possible, or maybe we associate hearing impairment with infirmity in general. And no doubt there are those of us who fear that if hearing loss has occurred, senility can't be far behind.

The Emotional Impact of Hearing Loss

Of course when examined rationally, these fears are un-
founded. As you've seen in the previous chapters, hearing
loss is an equal-opportunity condition: It doesn't discriminate among age, race, or sex. Many people are hard of
hearing from the day they're born. Similarly, there's absolutely no correlation between hearing loss and intelligence. If you took someone with perfectly normal hearing
to a country where she didn't speak the language, would
she instantly lose a few IQ points? Of course not. Might
she feel stupid or frustrated because she wouldn't be able
to understand what people were saying to her? Undoubt-
edly. The same is true for people who are hearing impaired: Their native intelligence doesn't deteriorate along
with their hearing. (However, if they withdraw into a shell
and lose interest in their friends, families, work, or current events, they may unwittingly contribute to the illu-
sion that they're no longer as sharp as they used to be.)

But emotions aren't rational. They spring from another
part of ourselves—the part concerned with self-esteem,
with the ability to initiate and maintain relationships, and
with the desire to lead a full and interesting life. Hearing
loss is an emotional issue because it can affect all these
areas. For example,

*Sarah is a 33-year-old woman who lost 80 percent of her
hearing shortly after birth. She attended special schools
and has worn hearing aids most of her life; so she can
function fairly normally. Nevertheless, she has a distinct
speech impediment and often finds it difficult to understand what's said to her in a noisy environment, such as
a party or a crowded store. Sarah struggles daily with*

COPING WITH HEARING LOSS   79

these challenges and must remind herself constantly that the difficulties she encounters don't reflect on her. "Yet," she says, "it seems as if every time I confront my loss, remind myself that I'm still an okay person, and try to do my best, I meet another boulder, another sigh, another refusal to repeat a phrase, another lost punch line, another person who says, 'Never mind; it's not important.'"

Sarah's despair illustrates the uncertainty so many hearing-impaired people feel. They're never completely sure of what's being said and are often the targets of impatience or misunderstanding from the people they're talking to.

Reasons for Denial

For all these reasons, it's not surprising that denial is common among people who experience a hearing loss. Let's look at Charlie again.

He appeared to be quite sanguine about his retirement, and to a great extent he was. After all, he'd given many years to his company and deserved this time to enjoy life. Yet, on another level, Charlie was depressed. Retirement meant giving up a job he'd loved; it meant changing the routine he'd maintained for decades; it meant rarely or perhaps even never again seeing people he'd worked with for years. And on a more basic level, retirement meant getting old. To Charlie, losing his hearing only reinforced the fact that he was aging. So instead of saying to himself, "Maybe I should get my ears checked," he said to Anne, "Your mother's getting old" or "Why don't you speak up?" As communication became more difficult,

Charlie spent more time in front of the television, with the volume turned up so loud his wife, Rita, found it painful to listen to. She, and many other people, spoke to Charlie less and less because it became just too irritating to be interrupted with his incessant, "Huh? What? I can't understand you. . . . Speak up!"

For people with a hearing loss, it's often easier to withdraw than it is to brave the sighs, the lost punch lines, the refusals to repeat phrases which Sarah spoke of. And indeed, such incidents are painful for everyone, no matter how well adjusted they may be. But sometimes, people who are losing their hearing become so immersed in coping with that loss—or in the mental gymnastics required to deny its existence—that they forget that their hearing loss doesn't affect only them: It affects those around them, as well. Of course, some problems are normal at first. After a while, however, if individuals with a hearing impairment don't learn how to live with their condition, it could have a profound impact on those who must deal with them every day: family, coworkers, and friends.

Denial by Family and Friends

It's painful to watch a loved one develop an infirmity, but it's perhaps even worse to watch him or her become isolated and withdrawn. In an attempt to protect the hearing-impaired person from the kind of slights Sarah described, family members often try to remove him or her from as much outside contact as possible.

When Charlie and Rita eat in restaurants, Rita orders for both of them—sometimes without even asking Charlie what he wants. She's seen the annoyance on waiters' faces when he asks them to repeat, over and over, the daily specials or questions such as "How do you want that cooked?"

Sarah still has to remind her mother not to answer questions for her. Recently, they went shopping together. Sarah was looking at shoes when a salesman approached her and asked if she'd like to try on a pair. Before Sarah could respond, her mother said, "Oh, no, that's all right —she's just looking." As it turned out, Sarah had wanted to try on the shoes.

Efforts like these are well meaning, but their actual result is to remove the hearing-impaired person even more from the real world. In some cases, they may also prevent the person from truly accepting his or her hearing loss and developing ways of coping with it.

Sarah, of course, has long since acknowledged her hearing loss and has managed to live with it quite well. She's even developed a repertoire of gentle yet assertive responses for those times when her mother does try to do her talking for her.

But Charlie needs all the encouragement he can get to confront his hearing loss and receive help for it. His hearing loss is also exacerbating the tensions that already existed within his marriage: Remember that Charlie and Rita had very different expectations about the life they would lead after Charlie retired, and Rita had had some long-smoldering resentments about Charlie's lack of out-

*side interests. As Charlie became more and more with-
drawn due to his hearing loss, Rita became increasingly
disgusted. Interestingly, she never considered the fact
that he might be losing his hearing. For her, his isolation
was simply one more example of how "difficult" he was.
Ultimately, she left him to his own devices completely
and pursued a social life with her friends. Rita wasn't
being cruel; she simply didn't know how to express her
fear, frustration, and resentment in any other way.*

Might Rita have been engaging in some denial of her
own? Perhaps. It's just as important for family and friends
to accept a loved one's hearing loss. Such acceptance has
both emotional and practical value. If good communication with friends and family members is to be maintained,
those close to the hearing-impaired person will have to
learn to change their behavior in certain ways, as you'll
see a little later in this chapter. Those who cannot acknowledge the fact of a loved one's hearing loss may never
adapt to it and thus may unwittingly help reinforce that
person's feelings of helplessness and isolation.

Impact on Children and Family

It's hard for parents to stand by and watch a child struggle
with a hearing loss.

*Sarah remembers being teased about her hearing aid,
and one particularly nasty incident in the second grade
in which some children cornered her on the playground,
making fun of her speech and yelling, "Dummy! What's
that thing in your ear? Don't you hear right?" It's impor-*

tant to encourage hearing-impaired children to lead as normal a life as possible, but unfortunately, you can't shield them from all the world's cruelty or ignorance. Sarah's parents could only listen sympathetically, tell her that the other children were thoughtless, and remind her that no one is perfect: How many children in her class wore glasses or looked a little chubby? Because Sarah's parents acknowledged her hearing loss early on, they were able to take advantage of special counseling that prepared them, as well as anyone can ever be prepared, for these and other obstacles their daughter encountered during her childhood. Thanks to their vigilance, she grew up with her self-esteem relatively intact. Nevertheless, as shown earlier, she still has her moments of doubt and despair.

What happens if a child with normal hearing must grow up in a family in which another member is hard of hearing? If a deaf parent doesn't acknowledge something a child says, the child may feel rejected even if the parents have explained the reason why it sometimes appears that Mommy or Daddy may not be listening. Another danger is that because it's just easier to communicate with the parent who hears normally, the child may grow closer to that parent and rely on him or her to be the go-between.

Ten-year-old Roger, whose father lost much of his hearing in combat during the Vietnam War, came home ecstatic from his first Little League baseball game. Rushing into the living room, he saw his father. "Hi, Dad!" he yelled, then ran through the house until he found his mother. "Mom, we won! We won!" he exclaimed. Then he added, "Tell Dad my team won the game." Sandy, Roger's mother, was also guilty of occasional slips. For example, if she was going out shopping and had to leave Roger home with his father, she'd sometimes tell the boy, "Make sure you listen in case the phone rings and answer it for your father. It's too hard for him to hear over the phone."

Thus, a child experiences hearing loss differently from adults, whether that hearing loss is his (or hers) or a parent's. If the child himself is hearing impaired, he and his parents will need special training and equipment virtually from the day he's born (or from the day the hearing loss is detected) if he's to have any chance of a normal life. But a child's ego is fragile; he may feel embarrassed if he needs a hearing aid, if he has to attend special classes, or if his speech sounds funny to other kids. That's why it's important for his parents to acknowledge his hearing loss early, so the child himself can learn to live with it and recover from setbacks.

Tips for Parents of a Hearing-Impaired Child

If your child has a hearing problem, take your cue from Sarah's parents. Have her hearing evaluated as soon as possible. Then provide the child with everything she (or he) needs to help her develop her listening and speech skills as much as possible—hearing aids, speech therapy, special classes, and so on. In addition, work with your child at home. It's not enough for her to practice in class; she's got to learn how to communicate on an everyday, ordinary level. This will take a lot of work on your part, but it will be worth it. Finally, be supportive. You can't shield her from all the vicissitudes of life, but you can reassure her that she's a worthwhile human being regardless of how well or how poorly she hears—or does anything else, for that matter.

Children of Hearing-Impaired Parents

If the child hears normally but lives with a parent who is hearing impaired, he (or she) may feel abandoned by that person, despite the best explanations in the world. Or he may unwittingly abandon that parent himself, simply because it's easier to communicate with the other parent. And if the child is asked to take on extra responsibility, as Roger was when his mother asked him to answer the telephone for his father, he may feel resentful and put-upon. And perhaps worst of all, the child may believe that a parent's hearing loss is somehow his fault: "If I didn't yell so loud, maybe Daddy's hearing would be better." For all these reasons, *both* parents should make it their business to communicate with the child, giving him the opportunity to learn the best way of interacting with the parent who's hard of hearing. Equally important, the parents should let the child see them interact with each other, providing a model that the child can then build on.

From these stories, and perhaps from your own experience as well, you can see the profound impact a hearing loss has on the person affected and on everyone around him or her. As you'll see, it doesn't have to be that way, because so much help is available. But the hearing-impaired person will never be able to take advantage of it all until he or she can say, "I'm getting a little hard of

hearing; I should get help for it." If individuals with hearing loss and their families make some simple changes in
their behavior, life-styles, and methods of communication, their lives can improve even before they spend a
penny on special equipment.

What follows are some tips for living with a hearing
impairment. Practical *and* psychological suggestions are
included because sometimes all it takes is a few practical
measures to improve your hearing and communication
skills and thus the emotional quality of your life.

COPING WITH HEARING LOSS

If You're the One with the Hearing Loss

When considering any practical changes to help you hear
better, bear in mind that how you hear depends largely on
two factors: your proximity both to the sounds you want
to hear and to any interfering noise. The farther away you
are from something you really want to hear, like some
music on the radio, the less you'll be able to hear it. But
the closer you are to any unwanted noise like running
water or a television going in the next room, the more it
will interfere with the sounds you really want to listen to.

With this principle in mind, think about how you
might rearrange your environment to maximize your
ability to hear the things that are important to you. At
home, arrange the seating so that the people you want to
hear sit closest to your ear with the better hearing. Try to
place the television, stereo, or radio so that you're sitting

closest to it and as far away as possible from parts of the home that tend to be noisy, like the kitchen or bathroom.

This is also the time to start working on your listening skills. Listening is a lost art in this society, but when you have a hearing loss, the ability to listen well allows you to make the most of all the other help you get—and makes things a little easier for those around you, as well. Some tips for better listening follow.

Look at people while they're speaking.   You can infer a lot from a person's facial expression, body language, and general tone of voice, even if you don't catch every word he or she says.

Eliminate any source of competing noise.   It's just basic good manners to turn off the television or radio when someone's trying to make conversation, but when you have a hearing loss, these measures are essential to your full understanding of what's being said. Also try to hold the conversation in a part of the room or the house where you'll be distracted as little as possible by running water, flushing toilets, or noise from the outside. Anyone's hearing may be disrupted by noise from such disparate things as:

Microwave ovens

Traffic

Air conditioners or fans

Rustling newspapers

Wind

Dishwashers in operation or running water

Be honest about your limitations. Even if the person you're talking to knows you're hard of hearing, it's sometimes easy to forget, especially if you're having an interesting or heated discussion. If you've missed a point or didn't understand something, slow down. You might say something like, "I'm sorry—I didn't quite catch that. Would you mind repeating it?" or, "Could you speak a little slower? I want to make sure I hear everything you say." It's much easier to honor a request like that than it is to put up with someone who repeatedly stops conversations with, "Huh?" "What?" "Say that again?" "Why are you mumbling?" and so on. If you're at the bank or in a store, and you can't understand the teller or the salesperson, there's no shame in saying simply, "I'm a little hard of hearing. Could you repeat that please?"

Maximize your hearing ability at work. Ask to be moved to a different area if possible. If a different room isn't available, even a quiet corner or someplace near a wall is preferable to being in the middle of a busy, noisy station. With less background noise to interfere, you have a better chance of hearing and understanding what people say to you. You'll probably also find it easier to concentrate on your work.

Try to become more independent. Often, hearing-impaired people come to depend on family members to accompany them on visits to the doctor. Then the doctor will start addressing his or her questions and comments to the relative—because it's easier. However, for the person with the hearing loss, it might make him (or her) feel more independent and perhaps even boost his confidence to go to the doctor alone, so that the physician has to speak directly to him. However, before doing this, be sure the individual already has enough confidence and is comfortable enough with his hearing loss that he'll tell the doctor when he can't hear something.

Telephone Tips

If you find it difficult to use the telephone, here are some tips that might help.

Install a telephone in a quiet part of your home.   This will eliminate as much background noise as possible, at least on your end. Also, get into the habit of putting the telephone receiver to the ear that hears better.

Remove your hearing aid before using the phone.   Some people wear their hearing aid in the ear that hears better. If that's the case, you may actually hear someone on the telephone better if you take the aid off before using the phone, because the hearing aid may distort the voice coming over the telephone.

Living with a Hearing-Impaired Person

Communication depends on all parties involved, so if you live or work with someone who's hard of hearing, there are changes that you, too, can make to help that person participate more in what's going on around him or her.

Speak a bit more slowly and clearly than you might ordinarily.   If your voice tends to be high-pitched, try to speak in a slightly deeper tone. Speaking so you can be understood is probably the single most important thing you can do to improve your relationship with someone with a hearing loss.

Make sure the person realizes you're speaking to her. This may seem silly, but people with normal hearing often address other people who are preoccupied or whose backs are turned, assuming that they'll hear what's being said. But if the person you're talking to is hard of hearing, you can't make that assumption. So, first attract her attention to let her know you're speaking to her. A gentle touch on the shoulder, or perhaps a wave if she can see you coming, is a possible approach. Before you actually start speaking, move close to the person and face her; many hearing-impaired people have subconsciously learned to read lips, which enhances their understanding even if they wear a hearing aid. Next, speak slowly and distinctly, as described above. And finally, make sure the environment is conducive to good hearing. If the room is noisy for some reason, either wait until the source of the noise is gone (such as traffic on a street outside) or move to a place where it's quieter.

Make sure that the person has understood what you've said. If you know her very well, you may be able to tell just from the expression on her face or from her body language whether or not she's accurately heard what you've told her. If there's any doubt, ask her to repeat it back to you. Or ask her a question and see if the answer makes sense. Stop at any point you detect any uncertainty from the person with the hearing loss and ask her if she has any questions or if she's heard what you've said.

Be aware of your own body language and the tone of voice; make sure they match the content of what you're saying. As with lipreading, hearing-impaired people often depend on these features to provide information about what people are saying. Any discrepancy between what you're actually saying and the tone in which you're saying it, or the position of your body as you're saying it, can confuse someone who cannot hear well.

Don't shout! It may be tempting at times, but in fact shouting usually doesn't help someone with a hearing impairment, especially if the loss is mild. And as you saw in Chapter Two, it may even hurt; there are certain forms of hearing loss in which soft conversation is heard more easily than shouting.

Save really important matters for when you're both relaxed and in a quiet environment.   If your friend with the hearing impairment feels unhurried and at ease, she will find it much easier to listen to you and to be alert for all the little cues that enhance understanding, such as lipreading and body language. And you'll find it easier to be patient, to remember to speak slowly and distinctly, and to repeat anything that might not have been understood.

Just as it's easier to communicate when you're both at ease, it's harder to speak to someone when one or both of you are tired, ill, or under stress.   Save anything truly important for when you're feeling better, and take into account the fact that you're currently going through a difficult period.

Be honest with the hearing-impaired person. If you're not certain of the best way to communicate with her, say so. Tell her that if you ask her if she's heard you, or if she has any questions, or if she wants you to repeat what you've said, you're not trying to be patronizing—you just want to make sure she's heard you accurately. Tell her also to inform you as to what's helpful and what's not. For example, maybe it really does help when you lower your tone of voice a bit. Or perhaps she hears best when you face her, so she can see your expression and read your lips. Finally, make it clear that acknowledging her hearing loss does *not* mean that you think she's slowing down or getting senile. All it means is that one member of the family has developed a condition that requires some adjustments on everyone's part but that all of you can live with very well once those adjustments have been made.

Find an outlet for expressing your feelings. You may feel angry, frustrated, and perhaps even depressed at times, especially in the beginning. Fortunately, there are lots of support groups—for hearing-impaired people themselves and for their families—where everyone can air feelings without fear of hurting or angering someone they love. You'll find a list of some support groups in the final chapter of this book. *Use it!* Don't let anger or resentment build until you find yourself saying or doing something you'll later wish you hadn't.

For many people, hearing loss is a condition that must be grappled with emotionally before it can be treated clinically. This chapter has focused on those individuals, touching on the importance of acknowledging the hearing loss; on the ways the hearing-impaired person and his or her loved ones can make the environment more conducive to good communication; on the subtle ways in which one person's hearing loss can affect an entire family; and on the impact of hearing loss on a child.

It must be added that not everyone finds it hard to accept a hearing loss. Perhaps you've been reading this chapter in some perplexity, thinking, "Why are they turning it into such a big deal? I've never had most of these problems. I know I'm hard of hearing, and I just want to learn more about it." If that's the case for you, feel lucky that you've managed to avoid the problems discussed here. Remember, however, that coping with hearing loss presents a formidable challenge for many, many people—those with the hearing impairment and the people they love. For them, coming to grips with their condition is essential to availing themselves of the help that's available. In the next chapter, you'll learn about hearing aids and other assistive devices that help make life a little less silent.

SIX

HEARING AIDS, OTHER DEVICES, AND SURGERY

According to the International Hearing Society, more than 14 million people in the United States could benefit from the use of a hearing aid. However, only slightly more than 5 million people regularly use these devices. Thus, nearly two thirds of the people who could benefit from hearing aids don't use them. Often, this is due to the problems mentioned in Chapter Five: denial that the hearing loss exists or that it's as severe as it is, or the equation of a hearing impairment with mental impairment or encroaching senility.

Some people may be willing to use a hearing aid but don't know how to go about getting one or are convinced that a hearing aid won't help them. Indeed, many people wear hearing aids for a while and then discard them, finding the devices useless or uncomfortable. Almost always, these problems result from improper fitting or from using the wrong kind of aid; it's usually *not* because the person can't be helped. Finally, some people don't want to try hearing aids because they're deterred by the expense.

While this is a real concern, there are ways you can get around this problem.

To derive real benefit from a hearing aid, you must know what kinds of hearing aids are available and how to obtain the best fit—both to your ear(s) and to your needs. It's also helpful to know a little about the way they work, to keep your expectations realistic.

ABOUT HEARING AIDS

First of all, what *is* a hearing aid? How exactly does it aid your hearing? Think of a hearing aid as a small amplifier, because that's essentially what it does: It picks up sounds from the environment, amplifies them, and sends the amplified signal into your ear.

Basically, a hearing aid is a tiny electronic device that contains a microphone, a speaker, and an energy source (a battery) along with the amplifier. The microphone detects the sounds that then are amplified and sent to the eardrum through the speaker. Like any portable electronic item, the hearing aid requires a source of energy, which is provided by the battery. A hearing aid can't make sounds any clearer, but it can make them *louder*. Newer model hearing aids can also screen out background noise, amplify only certain frequencies, or mask tinnitus.

Hearing aids are sold by people called *hearing aid dispensers*. These individuals run certain tests and help you select the hearing aid that best suits your needs; sometimes the dispenser may be an audiologist, but that training isn't required. Some hearing aid dispensers run their own offices independently of any one doctor or audiologist, whereas some doctors' offices may have hearing aid dispensaries right there on the premises as a convenience for their patients. You aren't required to buy your hearing aid there, however, and if you think you can do better someplace else, by all means, go.

To determine if a hearing aid is suitable for you, an audiologist should first perform the basic hearing tests described in Chapter Three to identify the nature and degree of your hearing loss. Then he or she will conduct a *hearing aid evaluation test,* which, as the name implies, determines if you'll be able to benefit from a hearing aid, and if so, which kind. During the evaluation, which lasts 60 to 90 minutes, the audiologist will test your hearing with and without different kinds of hearing aids. Using that information, he or she will prescribe the aid that best meets your needs and may even refer you to a hearing aid dispenser. The audiologist will also give you some advice on the best way to use and care for the hearing aid.

Okay, now you're set: You just go to the hearing aid dispenser, pick out your hearing aid, and you're done. Right? Wrong. To fit and function properly, hearing aids must be custom-made for each client. A hearing aid that's too tight can make the ear swell and become infected. If it's too loose, it may hurt or fall off. To avoid these problems, the hearing aid dispenser makes a wax impression of your ear and sends it off to the factory, so they can make a hearing aid that melds to the contours of your ear as closely as possible.

Once you have your hearing aid, you'll probably be told to return to the audiologist for a *hearing aid measurement,* a test that uses a special machine to evaluate the hearing aid's function. This helps the audiologist ascertain that the hearing aid is indeed working properly.

Types of Hearing Aids

Hearing aids differ in style, depending on the wearer's needs: hearing loss in one or both ears, for example; the severity of the hearing loss; and in some cases, the person's age or level of manual dexterity. Finding a hearing aid that's right for you can be accomplished only through consultation with your doctor, audiologist, and hearing aid dispenser.

Here are brief descriptions of the hearing aids in most common use today.

All-in-Ear (AIE). Also called simply *in-the-ear hearing aids,* these devices fit entirely in your ear. They're built with special screens to protect you from extraneous noise like wind and to protect the mechanism itself from being plugged up with debris like earwax or dead skin.

Many people like AIE hearing aids because they don't interfere with eyeglasses and can be worn during strenuous physical activity, like a tennis game. Also, they're easy to manage for people who may have limited vision or manual dexterity. On the other hand, because the entire mechanism fits into the ear, it often makes the ear feel uncomfortably full. What's more, these aids may make it more difficult to use the telephone: You may have to teach yourself to hold the receiver differently, or you may find it easier to use a telephone amplifier if you often wear the aid while speaking on the phone (some people remove the hearing aid entirely to talk on the telephone). If you frequently develop dermatitis in the ear, or have a lot of earwax, an AIE aid probably isn't for you because, despite the protective screen, it may become plugged or damaged or contribute to the skin irritation. Finally, if appearance is important, you may want to consider another type of hearing aid because the AIE aids are relatively large and noticeable.

There's now another version of the AIE device available, known as a *low-profile hearing aid*. These are similar to AIE aids except that they have a plate attached in front to disguise the hearing aid's components. They're able to block out even more wind noise and are a little less obtrusive in appearance than AIE aids.

Canal Aids. If you'd prefer a hearing aid that's less noticeable, a canal aid may be for you. They're smaller and less visible than the AIE hearing aids, and they offer good sound quality. What's more, you don't have to worry about them when you use the telephone, and like the AIE devices, you can wear them during physical activity.

Unfortunately, however, the canal hearing aids have many drawbacks. First, they're suited only to people with mild to moderate hearing impairments; those with severe hearing loss won't benefit from these instruments. As with the AIE aids, canal aids are probably not best for people who are prone to dermatitis or excess moisture or wax in the ear canal. Also, not everyone's ear canal is large enough to accommodate these hearing aids; if the fit is too tight, your ear may feel full and you may experience some echoing of your voice when you speak. In addition, because these aids are so small and fragile, they're easy to drop, lose, or break, making them best for people whose manual dexterity is good. Finally, these aids are among the most expensive made, and they require more frequent visits to the audiologist or hearing aid dispenser for testing and adjustment.

Behind-the-Ear (BTE). If you have a fairly severe hearing loss, you may want to consider a BTE hearing aid. The microphone and tubes hang behind the ear and are connected to an ear mold containing the amplifier, which sits inside the ear. Often, BTE hearing aids are more sophisticated electronically than the other types, which makes them easier to adjust and more flexible to use—in fact, they're suitable for hearing losses ranging from mild to severe. In addition, BTE hearing aids are more powerful than other models and are comfortable, durable, and easy to use, making them suitable for people whose vision or manual dexterity might not be as good as they used to be.

As with anything else, however, BTE aids do have their drawbacks. If you're physically active, you may find them cumbersome. Occasionally, people complain that the BTE interferes with their eyeglasses, although this is by no means a common problem. When using the phone, you may have to learn to hold the receiver differently or to use a telephone amplifier. However, these and many other assistive devices were designed to be used with the BTE hearing aid, something you might want to consider if you think you'll be using many of them (some of which are discussed a bit later in this chapter).

Body Aids. Body hearing aids are probably the oldest type still in use; until the 1950s, they were the only kind available. With a body aid the microphone is fastened to your shirt or blouse; the sound it detects travels up a wire attaching the mike to a speaker in the ear mold.

These hearing aids are large and powerful, and therefore are recommended for people with profound hearing loss (who also won't be bothered by the rustling of their clothing the microphone will inevitably detect) and/or for individuals whose manual dexterity is really limited. Young children also occasionally benefit from body aids.

Eyeglass Aids. These hearing aids are built directly into the earpiece of your glasses, which at first may seem to make them extremely convenient and unobtrusive. But in fact, they're fraught with problems; for example, whenever you take off your glasses, you're also removing your hearing aid. And what happens if the glasses get lost or broken? Your hearing aid is gone as well. Similarly, every time you need a new prescription for your glasses, you have to make some arrangement for a hearing aid until you get your glasses back. All in all, combining one's glasses with a hearing aid may have seemed like a good idea at the time, but its actual value is dubious. Eyeglass aids are seldom prescribed anymore.

Bone Conduction Aids. Theoretically, these devices enhance hearing by applying vibrations to the bone behind the ear. They may help some people with profound hearing loss whose ear canals have been severely damaged, but these individuals must also become proficient at lipreading, because speech comprehension is very poor when compared with that obtained with other types of hearing aids. As with the eyeglass aids, bone conduction aids probably seemed better in theory than they did in practice. And as with the eyeglass aids, they're rarely recommended anymore.

Cros and Bicros Aids. People with functional hearing only in one ear are the chief beneficiaries of cros and bicros hearing aids. These aids are worn in each ear, with sound from the bad ear's side transmitted to the better ear, permitting you to hear what was said on your "bad" side. Cros aids are for people whose good ear needs no amplification; with them, sound coming from the bad side won't seem weaker. Bicros aids are for people whose better ear needs some amplification; so they serve the dual purpose of improving hearing in that ear and helping you hear what was said on the side of the worse ear.

How Many Hearing Aids?

You may have to decide if you want to wear a hearing aid in both ears or only in one. Most experts feel that if you've sustained a hearing loss in both ears, you should wear hearing aids in both ears. This will help maximize your understanding of speech, especially when you're in a crowded or noisy environment like a restaurant or auditorium. Sounds will seem clearer and stronger with two aids, and you'll be able to detect their location more easily. You may even be able to use visual cues more efficiently because you'll have a better idea of the sound's origin. In short, two hearing aids will more closely approximate normal hearing. If this has been recommended for you, take the advice.

Buying Smart

Hearing aids are fragile, expensive devices, ranging in price from $500 to as much as $2,000. It usually takes a few weeks or even more to learn how to use them for maximum benefit; often you may have to go back to the dispenser or audiologist several times for adjustment and more training. In addition, the people who buy hearing aids are often quite vulnerable—they may have come to terms with their hearing loss only reluctantly; they may be living on a fixed income and terrified at the thought of paying for a hearing aid; and/or they may be intimidated by the whole idea of using and caring for these little machines. For all these reasons, hearing aid buyers have, in the past, been prime targets for unscrupulous dealers who've been all too willing to take someone's money and sell him or her something worthless. Even the finest, most modern hearing aid in the world will be of no value if it proves too complicated or uncomfortable to use.

To protect consumers from situations like these, many states now have laws governing the warranties issued with hearing aids. In California, for example, you can use the hearing aid for 30 days before you decide if it's right for you. At the end of that time, you can return it either for a refund (the dispenser may be entitled to subtract a certain amount for his or her time and efforts) or for another hearing aid.

Remember, however, to keep your expectations realistic. Effective use of hearing aids depends on several factors, the first of which is your willingness to put in the time and effort it takes to use the instrument properly. You might also enlist the aid of those closest to you, asking them to speak while standing at various distances and angles from you, so you can get an idea of the hearing aid's power and range. Try it out in different situations— home, work, stores, restaurants, and so on—to learn its limitations. You may discover that you may have to adjust it when going from a quiet to a noisy environment or to one in which there's likely to be background noise (such as outdoors in the park, where there might be wind, leaves rustling, and similar sounds). Practice taking it out and putting it in until you become proficient, and learn the best way to clean it and store it. Finally, remember that while a hearing aid can certainly help you hear better, it can't make your hearing perfectly normal; there'll always be a difference, which you must get used to. So if your state permits a trial period, take advantage of it. It's for an important cause.

A Note on Finances.   There's no denying it: Hearing aids are expensive. What's more, they're rarely covered by insurance. It's been estimated that 1.2 million Americans cannot afford the most basic hearing aid for their needs. And among those people who manage to "afford" one, many must part with a dismayingly large chunk of their budget or make do with a hearing aid that's really inadequate for their needs. What can you do?

One option is to try to make an agreement with the hearing aid dispenser. Ask if he or she will let you make a down payment and then pay the balance in installments. These individuals often deal with clients living on a fixed income, so such requests are not alien to them.

Some hearing aid dispensers accept credit cards. You could charge your hearing aid and then pay it off that way. This may not be the ideal option, but at least you won't have to worry about coming up with the entire cost all at once.

Finally, you might consider obtaining a used hearing aid. A Denver-based organization known as Hear Now has established a national hearing aid bank, to which people donate their used hearing aids. The aids are reconditioned and repaired, then given to needy individuals. Should you really need a hearing aid and find that you absolutely can't afford one, contact Hear Now (their address is given in the last chapter of this book) and learn how you can get one from them. And by the way, if *you* have an old hearing aid you can't use anymore, they'll be grateful for the donation.

OTHER ASSISTIVE DEVICES

Hearing aids are just the beginning: The list of *assistive devices* (defined as anything other than a hearing aid that's designed to help the hearing impaired) is so vast that a complete description could easily fill the rest of this book. In fact, some assistive devices may even be more helpful with everyday living than the most up-to-date hearing aid. For example, hearing aids aren't meant to be worn to bed. How do you know if the phone rings or your alarm clock goes off? Assistive devices exist to fill those needs. What about watching television? People often find their hearing aids distort sounds from the television set or just aren't powerful enough to allow them to hear everything. Or they have to turn up the volume so much it's unbearable to anyone else in the room. The right assistive device can help solve those problems. Need something to tell you when your car blinker is going? Or when the doorbell is ringing? There's a device for those functions. Want to hear the sermons on Sunday morning? Or a play on Saturday night? There's something out there for you, too.

What follows are descriptions of the most widely used assistive devices. If you don't find what you want in this list, contact one or more of the organizations listed in Chapter Seven for more complete information.

Telephone Devices

Perhaps one of the greatest challenges faced by someone with a hearing loss is using the telephone. As you've seen, many hearing aids are too cumbersome to use comfortably with the telephone, so people wind up taking them off. And anyway, they often find they hear better without the aid, because hearing aids often distort voices on the telephone. Other hearing-impaired people, however, discover that voices just don't sound loud enough, or they come across distorted, when heard on a telephone receiver. Several telephone devices have been developed to help solve these problems.

Telecommunication Device for the Deaf (TDD). These instruments allow people with profound or complete hearing loss to communicate by telephone. To use a TDD, however, you have to be sure the person you're calling has one, too. The caller puts the receiver on a machine resembling a typewriter and types what he or she wants to say. The device converts the typed words into phone signals and converts them back into words at the other end. The other person's machine then prints them out. TDD equipment costs $250 to $550 for an individual set, and should be available through most local phone companies.

Fax Machines. As an alternative to the TDD, you might consider buying or leasing a facsimile, or fax, machine. These machines resemble telephones but have a slot through which you feed a piece of paper on which you've written or typed what you want to say. You then simply dial the receiving party's fax number, and the material you've written is transmitted and printed out on the other end. As with the TDD, the other person has to have a fax machine, too, but these are now standard office equipment, and home fax machines are becoming more and more accessible in design and cost. Available at most large electronics or office equipment stores, the better fax machines start at about $300 to $400, but prices are getting lower.

Ring Enhancers. Sometimes it's hard to hear the telephone ring, such as when you're in another room or if you're running water or an appliance like the vacuum. People who can't always hear the phone often find it helpful to equip it with a special signaling or alerting device. Some of these items simply make the sounds louder. If you have a large home, you might want to install these telephone ringers in every room (you can hook them up to one telephone and then put them in other rooms) so you'll be sure to hear the ring anywhere in the house.

If you're profoundly hard of hearing, if you want to make sure you'll know if the phone rings while you're asleep, or if you simply don't want the phone ringing in every room of the house, there are devices that offer silent signals—for example, a light that flashes when the phone rings. There's even a vibrating device you can put under your mattress or pillow—when the phone rings, it vibrates and wakes you up.

Amplifiers. If voices on the telephone simply don't sound loud enough, several types of telephone amplifying devices are available. One consists of a *volume controller* (also called a *telephone amplification device*) in the receiver, which can increase the volume of an incoming voice up to 30 percent. Many pay telephones are now equipped with these instruments. You can get one from your local telephone company, but they are expensive. Less expensive are amplifiers that plug into the receiver on one end, and the telephone itself on the other. These are available from some phone stores or hearing aid dispensers. Most of the devices described in the preceding paragraphs cost about $15 to $50.

There's also a device called a *T-switch* or *T-coil*, which is built directly into your hearing aid. The T-switch lets you change the volume from the phone by adjusting the volume on your hearing aid. Unfortunately, your telephone has to be specially equipped to respond to the T-switch, but once again, this can be arranged through your local phone company. Most hearing aids made today, especially behind-the-ear hearing aids, have T-switches. These devices are of greatest benefit to people with a severe hearing impairment.

Answering Machines.   You may also find a simple telephone answering machine of tremendous help. It relieves you of the burden of having to make sure all the right switches are adjusted as soon as the phone begins to ring. Instead, you can return the call at your leisure, when everything's set up or perhaps when the traffic in the street outside or the children playing on the sidewalk by your window have quieted down, so you can hear the conversation better. In some cases, you might even be able to anticipate what your conversation will be about, so you can listen for certain key words or phrases.

Similarly, some hearing-impaired people find it helpful to record telephone conversations, or at least those they have reason to believe will be important—a conversation with a lawyer or a banker, for example. Even if your phone is equipped with assistive devices, you might want to consider an answering machine just for your peace of mind, so you can play the conversation back as many times as needed to make sure you got everything right.

Group Listening Systems

A *group listening system* is anything that improves the hearing of more than one person at a time in a public forum such as a theater or a church.

FM Wireless Systems. These devices consist of a small, wireless, battery-operated FM microphone placed near the source of the sound, such as a priest giving a sermon, so it can transmit the sound to a tiny radio equipped with earphones. This arrangement affords high-quality transmission with less interference from background noise, and you can use it with or without a hearing aid. You can also use it individually, as for watching television.

Audio Loops. Audio loops work best for people whose hearing aids are equipped with T-switches. The person speaking wears a special microphone, which converts the sound of his or her voice into an electromagnetic signal. This signal is then picked up and transmitted by wires installed around the floor or walls of the room. The T-switch in the hearing aid can convert the electromagnetic signals back into sound waves so you can hear. People who don't wear hearing aids or whose aids lack T-switches can use special earphones that convert the signal into sound.

Many schools, theaters, and other public meeting places are now equipped with audio loops for the hearing impaired. The only drawback is that you have to sit within the "loop" circumscribed by the wires in order to hear the sound.

Infrared Systems. Sound signals coming from a transmitter are converted into infrared (lying outside the visible light spectrum) light beams, which carry the sound from the transmitter to a headset that looks like a doctor's stethoscope. The headset then converts the beams of light back into sound signals, which you hear. These systems are easy to install and offer good-quality sound, but their range is limited, and the light beams can't pass through obstructions such as walls; they also can't travel around corners.

Television Aids

As mentioned earlier in this chapter, the biggest problem when watching television is that when it's loud enough for the hearing-impaired person to hear, it's usually too loud for anyone else in the room to tolerate. That's where these devices come in. You can buy special earphones that connect to the television (most sets made today have a jack for earphones) but don't cut off the sound for other people. Thus, you can hear the television without interference from background noise or from a more comfortable visual distance. If you're going to invest in these earphones, try to find a pair equipped with its own volume control. You may be able to find these devices in electronics stores such as Radio Shack.

If you're handy, you might be able to hook up your own little speaker to the television, sort of like an extra speaker attached to a stereo. Then you can put the speaker in a position where you can best hear it. These devices are, for some reason, difficult to find in stores, so the best solution is to buy an ordinary, small stereo speaker and wire it so that it can connect to the television. Also, don't forget to connect it so that the regular volume control is unaffected for those who watch with you.

Closed-caption Devices.   Closed-caption (CC) devices, which attach to the television, display what the people on television are saying in the form of a subtitle that appears on the television screen. They don't interfere with the reception for those who hear normally. CC devices can be used only with programs broadcast especially for them (look for the little *CC* symbol on your television screen when a program first comes on); fortunately, most prime-time network entertainment and news programs are now accessible. And if you're thinking of buying a new television, you may want to wait until after July 1993: That's when the Decoder Circuitry Act goes into effect, requiring all television sets 13 inches or larger made in the United States after that date to have built-in captioning decoder circuitry, so you won't have to obtain a separate decoding unit.

Other Devices

If you need an alarm clock to wake you in the morning, or something to tell you when the doorbell's ringing, special signaling devices can perform these tasks. They function like the devices that tell you when the phone's ringing— by flashing a light when someone's at the door or by vibrating under your mattress or pillow when it's time to get up. Similar instruments can alert you when your baby's crying or help you use an appliance like the microwave oven. And what happens if you can't hear the turn signals in your car? You may not realize it if they don't go on when you want them to, or when you forget to turn them off. Now you can install a special signal device that emits high-pitched beeps audible even to people with very severe hearing loss; usually, you can hear them even if you don't wear a hearing aid.

Hearing-Ear Dogs

Since 1977, an Oregon-based organization known as Dogs for the Deaf has been rescuing puppies from pounds and training them to be helpers and companions to people who are completely deaf or profoundly hearing impaired. The dogs perform many of the duties performed by the assistive devices described above: They can tell you when the phone's ringing or someone's at the door, when the baby's crying, when the oven timer's going, or even when the smoke detector signals—all for a pat on the head and some food.

Actually, of course, it's more complicated than that. The dogs undergo a four- to six-month training program and are placed in a home only after the would-be owner is screened by the organization's staff. Once the dog is delivered, a trainer spends about a week with the recipient, teaching him or her the special hand signals that the dog has learned. Following the placement, the recipient must report regularly on the dog's progress.

These dogs aren't for everybody, but they have made a wonderful difference in many people's lives. If you'd like more information, contact Dogs for the Deaf at the address or phone number given in Chapter Seven.

SURGERY AND IMPLANTS

So far, you've seen that for hearing losses caused by infections or other medical conditions, the doctor can prescribe medication to resolve the condition and, it is to be hoped, bring your hearing back to normal. Sometimes, it's even simpler than that—removing some earwax or a foreign body is all that's necessary. In other cases, however, the lost hearing can never be restored; the best you can hope for is to prevent or at least delay any further hearing loss. Even in these instances, however, much help is available in terms of hearing aids and assistive devices.

Doctors do, however, have another weapon in their arsenal that might help someone with a hearing loss: surgery. Surgical techniques developed over the last 50 years represent possibly the most important advance in treatment for the hearing impaired, particularly if certain ear structures have been destroyed by infection or otosclerosis. Some of the surgical techniques ear specialists are likely to use today are described below.

Tympanoplasty

When infection has damaged or destroyed the three ossi-cles (the hammer, anvil, and stirrup), doctors may per-form a *tympanoplasty* to repair or even replace the dam-aged bones. The procedure can be performed in the doctor's office, under local anesthesia, with the doctor simply inserting instruments into the ear canal. A slightly more complicated procedure permits the repair of a dam-aged eardrum at the same time. In those cases, the doctor sometimes has to administer general anesthesia, and you'll probably have to spend a night in the hospital. Usu-ally, you can return to work after seven to ten days, and healing should be complete within about eight weeks. However, it may take several months more for your hear-ing to return to normal.

Myringoplasty

Myringoplasty refers to eardrum repair alone. With the patient under local anesthesia, the doctor fixes a perfo-rated eardrum with a bit of tissue taken from elsewhere in the ear. This seals the middle ear and helps restore hear-ing. Most people spend one night in the hospital and re-turn to work within a week; healing is complete and hear-ing is restored within six weeks.

Myringotomy Tube. As mentioned in Chapter Four, in the discussion on otitis media, if there's some residual infection or fluid left in the middle ear, the doctor may insert a tiny tube into the eardrum to allow the fluid to drain. These tubes usually stay in place with no trouble, eventually falling out when the eardrum heals over. Occasionally, however, they may cause an infection. You should suspect an infection if your ear suddenly starts draining from a tube that was inserted some time ago. In these cases, the doctor will most likely prescribe antibiotics and tell you to keep your ear dry.

Mastoid Surgery

Sometimes an infection may become so severe it spreads to the mastoid bone itself. Doctors can sometimes repair this bone damage by taking some bone and fat from behind the ear and filling in the mastoid cavity caused by the infection. If it's needed, the doctor will also repair the eardrum and even rebuild the ear canal. Every effort is made to restore hearing during this operation, but sometimes patients have to return once more, for a tympanoplasty.

Mastoid surgery is performed under general anesthesia but, as with the other types of surgery described here, requires only one night in the hospital. You can usually return to work within a week or two, and healing should be complete within about four months.

Cochlear Implants

A cochlear implant consists of a receiver/stimulator and an electrode array (a set of 22 tiny electrode bands packaged together) implanted in the inner ear. External components—including a microphone (to pick up sound), a speech processor (to convert the sound into an electrical signal), and a transmitter (to transmit the signal to the receiver)—activate the implanted parts. The transmitter conveys sound signals across the skin to the implanted receiver/stimulator, which converts the signals into electrical signals to be detected by the electrode array. The electrodes, in turn, stimulate different eighth nerve (hearing nerve) fibers, which send the messages on to the brain.

Cochlear implants were designed for people with complete nerve deafness. These individuals cannot wear hearing aids because hearing aids amplify sound impulses that the eighth nerve then carries to the brain for interpretation. If the eighth nerve isn't functioning for some reason, you won't be able to make sense of a sound, no matter how loud it is. So while a hearing aid makes sound louder, a cochlear implant transforms that sound into usable signals.

The best candidates for cochlear implants are people who lack useful hearing in both ears now but who were once able to hear well enough to develop some language skills. Also, they should have no serious health or medical problems, because the implant requires two to three hours of surgery under general anesthesia. There's no age limit; children as young as two and people in their seventies and eighties have received cochlear implants with no problem. The time to consider a cochlear implant is when you find you can no longer understand speech, even with a hearing aid; you may be able to hear voices or other sounds, but you can't distinguish the words those voices are saying unless you read lips. In short, if you can't understand speech with your eyes closed, you may be a candidate for a cochlear implant.

During surgery, the doctor inserts the electrode array

into the cochlea, and the receiver is placed on the mastoid bone behind the ear, just under the skin. The surgery isn't terribly painful, and when the skin is completely healed, the only evidence of the implant will be a small bump. You'll probably stay in the hospital one or two nights. The risks of surgery include:

Numbness of the scalp or ear

Possible injury to, or stimulation of, the facial nerve

Distortions in taste perception

Dizziness

Infection

However, these are rare and usually resolve quickly.

Once the internal components are in place, the external components can be fitted: the microphone, which sits behind the ear and resembles a behind-the-ear hearing aid; the speech processor, connected by wires to the microphone and hidden under the clothes; and the transmitting coil, connected to the processor by another microphone and hooked up to the receiver under the skin. This arrangement may take some getting used to, but most people will probably think you're wearing some kind of hearing aid—which, in a way, you are.

It's important to keep in mind that these devices don't restore hearing to normal. In fact, it takes up to nine months to adjust to them, although the people who have the implants say it's worth it. They're able to distinguish one sound from another, such as a knock at the door, the telephone's ring, a car horn beeping, and music. Cochlear implants also help recipients modulate their own voices. What's perhaps most important, however, is that you can once again understand what others are saying. Voices may sound funny at first (implantees describe other people as sounding like robots, Donald Duck, or Alvin the Chipmunk), but you'll get used to that. More than 90 percent of all implantees find that their lipreading abilities improve, and over half are able to understand at least 30 percent of what's said to them without lipreading. In fact, virtually everyone who receives a cochlear implant derives some benefit, although it's important to keep one's expectations realistic.

Cochlear implants represent an enormous stride in help for the hearing impaired, because they permit people who once were completely nerve deaf to hear *something*. What's more, technical improvements are being made all the time to afford implantees even better perception of speech, music, and other sounds. However, as you've seen, these devices still have their drawbacks. And they're very expensive: Prices average from $25,000 to $35,000 for the complete procedure. Fortunately, some insurance policies now cover at least part of that cost. At the moment, only a few thousand people in the world have cochlear implants, but as technology improves and prices come down, many thousands more will probably take advantage of this new technology.

Living with a hearing impairment isn't easy, and if you've suffered a permanent hearing loss, there's still nothing yet on the market that can restore your hearing to normal. Nevertheless, in this book we've tried to show you the many ways in which medicine and technology have tried to anticipate your needs. And research is ongoing continually. As improvements in hearing aids, cochlear implants, and assistive devices occur, they'll come closer and closer to offering normal hearing—perhaps even *better* than normal: They'll let you hear softer sounds, more clearly, and with less distracting background noise than many people who still rely solely on what nature gave them.

Why is research for the hearing impaired so active? Support and advocacy groups for the deaf and hearing impaired are well organized and have made the needs of their members clear. But there's more to it than that. Researchers obviously take the problems associated with hearing loss very seriously, and that could in large part be due to the fact that hearing loss is nearly ubiquitous in our society. So the important thing to remember is this: Whether it's you or a loved one who has the hearing loss, you're not alone. Hearing impairment affects millions of people and indirectly touches the lives of millions more. It doesn't mean you're getting senile or losing your grip; it simply means you've got a condition that needs attention. Think of your children's or grandchildren's voices; think of the music you love or any other sound you hold dear. Let that be your incentive to have your hearing checked *now*.

SEVEN

FOR MORE HELP

Perhaps, after reading this book, you've still got some questions. Maybe you've heard of a rare condition that wasn't mentioned, or perhaps you'd like to know more about the research that's being done on such disparate—yet related—topics as noise, hearing aids, or sign language. Or maybe you'd like to find a support group, either for people who are hearing impaired or for those who love and live with them.

What follows is a list of places that can either provide you with the information you're looking for or direct you to the proper source for it. In fact, this is really just a partial list: A complete tally could easily double the length of this book. If you've got a question, no matter how minute or esoteric it might appear, there's probably a support group, research organization, or government office somewhere that's looking at that very problem. Here are some that are most likely to be of help:

Alexander Graham Bell Association for the Deaf (AGB)
3417 Volta Place, NW

Washington, DC 20007
Telephone/TDD: (202) 337-5220

AGB is committed to speech education for hearing-impaired people and will disseminate information to anyone interested.

American Academy of Audiology (AAA)
6565 Fannin Street, Suite NA 200
Houston, TX 77030-2707
Telephone/TDD: (713) 798-3429

AAA is a professional organization for audiologists.

American Academy of Otolaryngology—Head and Neck
   Surgery (AAO-HNS)
One Prince Street
Alexandria, VA 22314
Telephone (voice only): (703) 836-4444

This organization promotes the art and science of medicine related to otolaryngology—head and neck surgery. Among the services it provides are continuing medical education courses and publications, such as free patient leaflets related to problems of the ears, nose, throat, head, and neck region. AAO-HNS can also refer you to a specialist in your part of the country.

American Deafness and Rehabilitation Association
(ADARA)
PO Box 251554
Little Rock, AR 72225
Telephone/TDD: (501) 663-7074

A membership organization and network that promotes, develops, and expands services, research, and legislation for deaf people. The American Society of Deaf Social Workers has reorganized as the Social Work section of ADARA.

American Hearing Research Foundation (AHRF)
55 East Washington Street, Suite 2022
Chicago, IL 60602
Telephone (voice only): (312) 726-9670

The AHRF supports medical research and education into the causes, prevention, and cure of deafness, impaired hearing, and balance disorders.

American Society for Deaf Children (ASDC)
814 Thayer Avenue
Silver Spring, MD 20910
Telephone/TDD: (301) 585-5400
Toll-free: (800) 942-ASDC

This membership organization provides information and support to parents and families with children who are deaf or hearing impaired.

American Tinnitus Association (ATA)
PO Box 5
Portland, OR 97207
Telephone (voice only): (503) 248-9985

The ATA provides education, information, and telephone counseling about tinnitus and self-help support.

Better Hearing Institute (BHI)
PO Box 1840
Washington, DC 20013
Telephone (voice only): (703) 642-0580

A nonprofit educational organization dedicated to informing hearing-impaired people, their friends and relatives, and the general public about hearing loss and available medical, surgical, and amplification assistance.

Boys Town National Research Center
555 North 30th Street
Omaha, NE 68131
Telephone (voice): (402) 498-6511; (TDD): (402) 498-6543

The Boys Town National Research Hospital specializes in communication disorders in children. It operates the National Research Register for Hereditary Hearing Loss, a clearinghouse for families interested in research on hereditary hearing loss. It also informs families of new research projects applicable to them and updates all families on the progress of ongoing research via its newsletter.

The Caption Center (CC)
125 Western Avenue
Boston, MA 02134
Telephone/TDD: (617) 492-9225

A nonprofit service of the WGBH Educational Foundation —WGBH is Boston's public television station—and the world's first television captioning agency. Produces captions for every segment of the entertainment and advertising industries and offers to clients an array of services, including off-line captions, real-time captions, and open captions. Development of software programs enables agencies and schools to caption their own programs and events.

Deafness Research Foundation (DRF)
9 East 38th Street
New York, NY 10016
Telephone (voice): (212) 684-6556; (TDD): (212) 284-6559

A voluntary health organization that provides grants for fellowships, symposia, and research into causes, treatment, and prevention of all ear disorders. The DRF also provides information and referral services.

Dogs for the Deaf, Inc.
10175 Wheeler Road
Central Point, OR 97502
Telephone/TDD: (503) 826-9220

Dogs for the Deaf rescues dogs from animal shelters and trains them to help hearing-impaired people. The animals are placed in approved homes free of charge, and organization staff members stay in touch to provide further training and other assistance when needed.

Ear Foundation (EF)
2000 Church Street, Box 111
Nashville, TN 37236
Telephone (voice): (615) 329-7807; (TDD): (615) 329-7809

A national, not-for-profit organization committed to leading the effort for better hearing and balance through public and professional education programs, support services, and applied research. An information resource for hearing-impaired people and the organizations that serve them. Also administers the Ménière's Network, a national network of patient support groups that provide people with the opportunity to share experiences and coping strategies.

Gallaudet University (GU)
800 Florida Avenue, NE
Washington, DC 20002-3695
Telephone/TDD: (202) 651-5000

Gallaudet University is a private, multipurpose educational institution and resource center that serves deaf and hard-of-hearing people around the world through a full range of academic, research, and public service programs. The university is committed to development of the intellect; to research aimed at improving the lives of deaf and hard-of-hearing people; and to service to them, their families and friends, and the professionals who work with them. The university also administers the National Information Center on Deafness.

Hearing Education and Awareness for Rockers (HEAR)
PO Box 460847
San Francisco, CA 94146
Telephone (voice only): (415) 441-9081
24-hour hotline: (415) 773-9590

HEAR operates a 24-hour hotline to provide information, assistance, and hearing screening appointments for those with hearing difficulties. Other HEAR activities include educational programs to educate young musicians and the consumer about the dangers of excessive sound levels.

Hearing Industries Association (HIA)
1255 Twenty-third Street NW
Washington, DC 20037-1174
Telephone (voice only): (202) 833-1411

The HIA represents firms that manufacture or distribute hearing aids, hearing health care products, and components. The HIA was established to increase the appropriate use of hearing aids by individuals with hearing losses who can benefit from amplification; to expand public knowledge of the role of hearing aids in improving the quality of life for the millions of hearing-impaired Americans; to work constructively with government, consumer leaders, and professional organizations to improve the health care system; and to conduct research and complete statistics reflecting the growth of the hearing aid industry.

Hear Now
4001 South Magnolia Way
Denver, CO 80237
Telephone (voice only): (303) 758-4919

Hear Now has a hearing aid bank for which the organization recycles used hearing aids for use by people who cannot afford new hearing aids.

House Ear Institute (HEI)
2100 West Third Street
Los Angeles, CA 90057
Telephone (voice): (213) 483-4431; (TDD): (213) 484-2642

A nonprofit organization that conducts research and provides information on hearing and balance disorders. The

Center for Deaf Children, a section of HEI, does evaluation and therapy.

John Tracy Clinic (JTC)
806 West Adams Boulevard
Los Angeles, CA 90007
Telephone (voice): (213) 748-5481
(TDD): (213) 747-2924
Toll-free: (800) 522-4582

Provides free diagnostic, habilitative, and educational services to preschool deaf children and their families through on-site services and to preschool deaf and deaf-blind children through worldwide correspondence courses in English and Spanish.

National Association of the Deaf (NAD)
814 Thayer Avenue
Silver Spring, MD 20910
Telephone (voice): (301) 587-1788; (TDD): (301) 587-1789

The NAD is an organization committed to improving the quality of products and services for deaf and hard-of-hearing people and a legislative advocate for equal access to communication and employment opportunities.

National Captioning Institute (NCI)
5203 Leesburg Pike, 15th Floor
Falls Church, VA 22041
Telephone/TDD: (703) 998-2400

Provides closed-captioning service for television networks, program producers, cablecasters, producers of home entertainment videocassettes, advertisers, and other organizations in the federal and private sectors. Additionally, distributes TeleCaption decoders to retailers around the country.

National Institute on Deafness and Other
  Communication Disorders (NIDCD) Clearinghouse
National Institutes of Health
PO Box 3777
Washington, DC 20013-7777
Telephone: (301) 496-7243

The NIDCD Clearinghouse was created in 1991 to collect and disseminate information on normal and disordered communication processes including diseases affecting hearing, balance, smell, taste, voice, speech, and language. The clearinghouse will make this information available to health professionals, patients, educators, industry, and the general public.

National Rehabilitation Information Center (NARIC)
8455 Colesville Road, Suite 935
Silver Spring, MD 20910
Telephone/TDD: (301) 588-9284
Toll-free: (800) 34-NARIC

A rehabilitation information service and research library that provides reference, research, and referral services; conducts custom data-base searches; publishes a quarterly newsletter; and disseminates rehabilitation-related information. NARIC has a data base, REHABDATA, which is a computerized listing of rehabilitation literature.

Self Help for Hard of Hearing People, Inc. (SHHH)
7800 Wisconsin Avenue

Bethesda, MD 20814   ·
Telephone (voice): (301) 657-2248; (TDD): (301) 657-2249

SHHH is a volunteer, international organization of hard-of-hearing people, their relatives, and friends. It is a non-profit, nonsectarian educational organization devoted to the welfare and interests of those who cannot hear well but are committed to participating in the hearing world.

Telecommunications for the Deaf, Inc. (TDI)
814 Thayer Avenue
Silver Spring, MD 20910
Telephone (voice): (301) 589-3786; (TDD): (301) 589-3006

A TCC/PC consumer-oriented organization that sells caption decoders and directories for deaf people. Supports legislation and advocates the use of TDDs, ASCII code, Emergency Access (911), telecaptioning, and visual alerting systems in the public, private, and government sectors.

TRIPOD
2901 North Keystone Street
Burbank, CA 91504
Telephone/TDD: (818) 972-2080
National toll-free: (800) 352-8888
California Grapevine: (800) 2-TRIPOD

Provides a national toll-free hotline for parents and individuals wanting information about raising and educating deaf children. TRIPOD operates a parent-infant-toddler program, Montessori preschool, and an elementary mainstream program for hearing-impaired children.

Very Special Arts, International (VSA)
1331 F Street NW, Suite 800
Washington, DC 20004
Telephone (voice): (202) 628-2800; (TDD): (202) 737-0645

VSA is a nonprofit organization that has helped bring children, youth, and adults with disabilities a special experience by creating and promoting year-round programs for them in drama, music, dance, and the visual arts. VSA is authorized by the United States Congress as the nation's coordinating agency for arts programs by, for, and with individuals who are disabled. Very Special Arts is composed of professionals and volunteers from a great variety of sources: business, education, the arts, media, and disabled citizens' groups, among others.

Vestibular Disorders Association of America
1015 NW 22nd Avenue, D230
Portland, OR 97120-3079
Telephone (voice only): (503) 229-7705

A nonprofit organization established exclusively to provide information and support for people with vestibular disorders and to develop awareness of the issues surrounding these disorders.

GLOSSARY

acoustic nerve   The cranial nerve concerned with hearing and balance. Also called the eighth nerve or eighth cranial nerve.

acoustic neuroma   A benign tumor arising from the acoustic nerve. Symptoms include loss of hearing and/or balance, tinnitus, facial numbness, and pain.

anvil   One of the three bones in the middle ear that help transmit sound waves from the outer ear to the cochlea and, ultimately, to the brain.

audiogram   A graph drawn by an audiologist depicting someone's ability to hear sounds at different frequencies.

audiologist   Someone trained in the science of audiology, who can administer hearing tests and helps in the rehabilitation of hearing-impaired people.

audiology   The study of hearing, especially hearing impairments that cannot be corrected through surgery or medicine.

auditory brain stem response audiometry   A hearing test designed to measure the ability of certain nerves to respond to sound. This test is most often performed on babies and other people who cannot communicate for some reason.

auricle The outer portion of the ear. Also called the pinna.

benign paroxysmal positional vertigo (BPPV) Vertigo that occurs when someone is sitting or lying down, thought to be caused by crystals settling in the jellylike fluid of the vestibular apparatus in the inner ear.

binaural hearing The phenomenon of hearing with both ears.

bone conduction The conduction of sound waves through reverberations of the mastoid bone to the inner ear.

central hearing loss Hearing loss that results from injury or illness to the nerves or portion of the brain concerned with hearing.

cerumen Earwax.

cochlea The major organ of the inner ear; it is shaped like a snail's shell and contains the organ of Corti, from which eighth nerve fibers actually send hearing signals to the brain. Also contains the vestibular apparatus, important in the control of balance.

conductive hearing loss Hearing loss caused by a problem in the outer or middle ear, resulting in the inability of sound to be conducted to the inner ear.

congenital hearing loss Hearing loss that is present from birth; it may or may not be hereditary.

cycles per second (cps) The measurement of frequency, or a sound's pitch.

decibel (db) The measurement of volume, or loudness.

dermatitis Any irritation of the skin. Some people are prone to dermatitis in the ear canal; excessive scratching may cause the canal to swell and may lead to conductive hearing loss.

ear canal   Part of the outer ear; the canal leading from the auricle to the eardrum.

eighth nerve   The cranial nerve concerned with hearing and balance; also called the acoustic nerve.

electrocochleography   A test of hearing nerve and inner ear function.

electronystagmography   A way of measuring the function of the vestibular apparatus by squirting cold water into the ear and watching the person's corresponding eye movements.

eustachian tube   The tube running from the nasal cavity to the middle ear, which helps maintain sinus and middle ear pressure.

frequency   A way of describing a sound's pitch. High-pitched sounds are high-frequency sounds; low-pitched sounds are low-frequency sounds.

group listening system   Equipment used to enhance the hearing of more than one person in public places such as churches or theaters.

hammer   One of the three bones in the middle ear that help transmit sound waves from the outer ear to the cochlea and, ultimately, to the brain.

hearing aid dispenser   A person who is specially trained to fit, test, and sell hearing aids.

Hertz (Hz)   A measurement of frequency; 1 Hz equals 1 cps (cycle per second).

impedance audiometry   A test that measures a person's ability to hear sound waves transmitted through bone, as opposed to those borne by sound.

inner ear   That part of the ear beginning with the oval window, consisting of the cochlea (including the vestibular apparatus). It is from the inner ear that sound signals are actually transmitted to the brain. Also concerned with the maintenance of balance.

labyrinthitis A viral infection of part of the vestibular canal, which may cause vertigo.

mastoid bone The bone in which the entire ear mechanism is housed. Part of a larger bone called the temporal bone.

mastoiditis Inflammation of the mastoid bone.

Ménière's disease A condition resulting from fluid buildup in the inner ear, leading to episodes of hearing loss, tinnitus, and vertigo.

middle ear That portion of the ear beginning at the eardrum, consisting of the ossicles (hammer, anvil, and stirrup), and bordered on the other side by the oval window. Helps concentrate and transmit sound waves to the inner ear. Also contains the eustachian tube, which helps maintain sinus and middle ear pressure.

mixed hearing loss Hearing loss resulting from both conductive and sensorineural impairment.

myringoplasty A surgical procedure for repairing a damaged eardrum.

nystagmus Rapid eye movements. In this book, the word *nystagmus* pertains to the eye movements associated with the function of the ear's balance mechanism.

organ of Corti Located in the cochlea, the organ containing the hair cells that actually transmit sound waves from the ear to the eighth nerve and the brain.

ossicles The collective name for the three bones of the middle ear: the hammer, anvil, and stirrup.

otitis externa Infection of the outer ear.

otitis media Infection of the middle ear.

otolaryngologist   A doctor who specializes in treating diseases of the ear, nose, and throat.

otologist   A doctor who specializes in treating diseases of the ear.

otology   The branch of medicine concentrating on diseases of the ear.

otorhinolaryngologist   A doctor who specializes in treating diseases of the ear, nose, and throat.

otosclerosis   A condition characterized by the formation of spongy bone around the stirrup in the middle ear, which prevents the stirrup from transmitting sound waves properly and thus causes conductive hearing loss.

outer ear   That portion of the ear consisting of the outer flap (the pinna, or auricle) and the ear canal. Bordered on the other side by the eardrum. Collects sound waves from the environment and directs them into the ear.

oval window   The membrane separating the middle ear from the inner ear. Its vibrations transmit sound into the cochlea.

pinna   The external portion of the ear. Also called the auricle.

presbycusis   Hearing loss associated with old age.

pure tone   A tone composed of one frequency only.

pure-tone hearing test   A test of someone's ability to hear tones of different frequencies.

semicircular canals   Part of the vestibular apparatus of the cochlea; help in maintaining balance.

sensorineural hearing loss   Hearing loss that results from a problem in the inner ear.

serous otitis media   A middle ear infection characterized by a discharge from the ear, due to fluid leakage from a perforated eardrum.

stirrup   One of the three bones in the middle ear that help transmit sound waves from the outer ear to the cochlea and, ultimately, to the brain.

temporal bone   The larger bone that contains the mastoid bone.

tinnitus   Ringing or buzzing in the ears.

tympanum   The eardrum; also called the tympanic membrane.

vertigo   The sensation of moving or spinning while actually sitting or lying still.

vestibular apparatus   The part of the cochlea concerned with the maintenance of balance.

vestibuloocular system   The system that coordinates vestibular apparatus function with eye movements to help maintain balance and to make quick adjustments in sudden changes of motion or position.

INDEX

Acoustic neuroma, 25

Age-related hearing loss, 24–25, 50–51

Air pressure, 10

Alcohol, 38, 48

Alexander Graham Bell Association for the Deaf (AGB), 119–120

Allergies, 53–54

All-in-Ear (AIE) hearing aids, 97–98

American Academy of Audiology (AAA), 120

American Academy of Otolaryngology-Head and Neck Surgery (AAO-HNS), 32, 36, 41, 120

American Acoustical Society, 64

American Deafness and Rehabilitation Association, 120–121

American Hearing Research Foundation (AHRF), 121

American Society for Deaf Children (ASDC), 121

American Tinnitus Association (ATA), 121

Amplifiers, 106–107

Answering machines, 107–108

Antibiotics, 25, 38, 44, 67, 69

Antihistamines, 44

Anvil, 3–4, 6, 14, 113

Aspirin, 25, 44

Assistive devices, 104–111

Audiogram, 45

Audiologists, 42–43

Audio loops, 108–109

Auditory brain stem response audiometry, 48–49

Auditory nerve, 6

Auditory training, 27

Auricle, 2–3

Background noise, 22, 26–27, 63, 87–89, 95, 102–103

Balance, 5, 6, 11, 12, 55

Balance tests, 47–48

Behind-the-Ear (BTE) hearing aids, 99

Benign paroxysmal positional
   vertigo (BPPV), 13
Better Hearing Institute (BHI),
   122
Bicros hearing aids, 100–101
Binaural hearing, 9
Body hearing aids, 99–100
Body language, 87, 91
Bone conduction, 22–23, 26
Bone conduction hearing aids,
   100
Bone conduction tests, 46
Bonine, 48
Boys Town National Research
   Center, 122
Brain, 6, 7, 28

Canal hearing aids, 98
Caption Center (CC), 122–123
Central hearing loss, 28
Cerumen (earwax), 3, 14, 19–20
Children, 14, 20, 32–33, 36–40,
   65–68, 70, 82–85
Chronic otitis media, 67–68
Closed-caption devices, 111
Cochlea, 4, 6, 11, 12, 15, 50, 59,
   69
Cochlear implants, 114–117
Conductive hearing loss, 18–23
Congenital hearing loss, 21
Consonants, 8–9, 17, 26, 27, 63
Cros hearing aids, 100–101
Cued speed, 27
Cycle, 8
Cycles per second (cps), 8

Deafness Research Foundation
   (DRF), 123
Decibels (db), 9, 17, 18, 61, 64

Denial of hearing loss, 77–82, 94
Dermatitis, 20
Dihydrostreptomycin, 44
Discharge, 18
Discomfort level, 45
Diuretics, 25
Dizziness, 11–13, 25, 31, 47, 48,
   53
Dogs, 111–112
Dogs for the Deaf, Inc., 112, 123
Dramamine, 48

Ear anatomy, 2–6
Ear canal, 3, 6, 14, 59
   obstruction in, 19–20
Ear care, 71–72
Eardrum, 3, 6, 14, 50, 66–67
   injuries to, 21, 70–71, 113–114
Ear Foundation (EF), 123–124
Ear pain, 18, 21, 31, 66, 68–69
Earwax, 3, 14, 19–20
Eczema, 20
Eighth cranial nerve, 6, 13, 25,
   55, 115
Electrocochleography, 48
Electronystagmography (ENG),
   47–48
Emotional impact of hearing
   loss, 75–93
Eustachian tube, 10–11, 20, 65
Eyeglass hearing aids, 100

Fax machines, 105–106
Flu, 25
Fluid, 4–6, 11–13, 21, 53, 54,
   66–67, 113–114
Flying, 10–11
FM wireless systems, 108
Foreign objects, 14, 20, 69–70

Frequency, 8, 9, 59, 63

Gallaudet University, 124
German measles, 24, 38
Group listening systems, 108–109

Hair cells, 4–6, 8, 11, 50, 59
Hammer, 3–4, 6, 14, 113
Hardening of the arteries, 15
Head injuries, 24, 38
Hearing, 1–15
Hearing aid dispensers, 95–96, 102, 103
Hearing aid evaluation test, 96
Hearing aids, 27, 52, 94–104
Hearing-ear dogs, 111–112
Hearing Education and Awareness for Rockers (HEAR), 124
Hearing-impaired parents, children of, 85–86
Hearing Industries Association (HIA), 125
Hearing loss
  age-related, 24–25, 50–51
  children and, 14, 20, 32–33, 36–40, 65–68, 70, 82–85
  common diagnoses of, 49–55
  emotional impact of, 75–93
  information sources, 119–129
  noise-induced, 24, 50, 51, 57–65, 72–73
  prevention of, 57–74
  selection of physician, 37, 41–43
  sensoineural, 6, 23–27
  signs of possible, 30–32
  surgery, 52, 54–55, 66, 112–117

tests, 32, 34–35, 43–49
types of, 16–28
Hearing specialists, 37, 41–42
Hear Now, 103–104, 125
Heart disease, 50
Hertz (Hz), 8, 44
High blood pressure, 50
High-risk jobs, 60–61, 64
Hospitals, 41–42
House Ear Institute (HEI), 125–126

Impedance audiometry, 46–47
Infants, 32, 36, 38–39
Infections, 14, 15, 20–21, 65–69, 71
Information sources, 119–129
Infrared systems, 109
Infrared (video) electronystagmography, 47
Inner ear, 4–6, 11–13, 15 (see also Hearing loss)
Insects, 14
Intelligence, 77, 78
International Hearing Society, 94

Johns Hopkins Hospital, 43
John Tracy Clinic (JTC), 126

Kanamycin, 44

Labyrinthitis, 69
Lipreading, 17, 27, 117
Low-profile hearing aid, 98

Massachusetts Eye and Ear Infirmary, 42
Mastoid bone, 22, 46, 66
Mastoiditis, 66, 67

Mastoid surgery, 114
Mayo Clinic, 42
Measles, 24
Medical history, 43–44
Ménière, Prosper, 53
Ménière's disease, 13, 15, 53–55
Meningitis, 25, 38, 67
Middle ear, 3–4, 6, 10, 14, 15
    (see also Hearing loss)
Mild hearing loss, 17
Mixed impairment, 27
Moderate hearing loss, 17
Mumps, 24
Myringoplasty, 113
Myringotomy tube, 113–114

Nasopharynx, 10
National Association for the Deaf
    (NAD), 126
National Captioning Institute
    (NCI), 126–127
National Institute on Deafness
    and Other Communication
    Disorders (NIDCD)
    Clearinghouse, 127
National Institutes of Health, 63,
    127
National Rehabilitation
    Information Center (NARIC),
    127
Neomycin, 44
Newborns, 33, 37–39
Noise-induced hearing loss
    (NIHL), 24, 50, 51, 57–65,
    72–73
Numbness, 25
Nystagmus, 12

Occupational Safety and Health
    Administration (OSHA), 64
Organ of Corti, 4–6, 8, 59
Ossicles, 3, 4, 10, 14, 50, 113
Otitis externa, 14, 68–69
Otitis media, 14, 20–21, 65–68
Otolaryngologists, 37, 41
Otologists, 19, 41
Otology, 37
Otorhinolaryngologists, 41
Otosclerosis, 14, 44, 51–52
Outer ear, 2–3, 14 (see also
    Hearing loss)
Oval window, 4, 51

Perforated eardrum, 21, 66–67,
    113
Permanent threshold shift (PTS),
    59, 60
Physician, selection of, 37, 41–43
Pinna, 2–3
Pregnancy, 24, 38, 52
Presbycusis, 24, 49–51
Prescription drugs, 25–26, 48
Profound hearing loss, 17
Pure-tone hearing test, 44–45

Quinine, 44

Ring enhancers, 106
Ringing in ears, 25, 27, 32, 53,
    95

Scarlet fever, 25
Seasickness remedies, 48
Self Help for Hard of Hearing
    People, Inc. (SHHH), 127–
    128
Semicircular canals, 11, 12, 15

Sensoineural hearing loss, 6, 23–27

Serous (perforated) otitis media, 14, 66–67

Severe hearing loss, 17

Sign language, 27

Sinuses, 20

Sound waves, 7–9

Speech hearing or discrimination test, 45

Speech retraining, 27

Startle reflex, 33, 39

Stirrup, 3–4, 6, 14, 51, 113

Streptomycin, 25, 44

Stress, 53

Sulfa drugs, 44

Support groups, 92

Surgery, 52, 54–55, 66, 112–117

Swimmer's ear, 68–69

Swimming, 20, 69, 72

Telecommunication Device for the Deaf (TDD), 105

Telecommunications for the Deaf, Inc. (TDI), 128

Telephone devices, 105–108

Telephone tips, 89, 97, 99

Television aids, 109–110

Temporal bone, 2, 22

Temporary threshold shift (TTS), 59, 60

Tests, 32, 34–35, 43–49

Tinnitus, 25, 27, 32, 53, 95

TRIPOD, 128

T-switch, 107–109

Tumors of the eighth nerve, 13, 25

Tympanoplasty, 113

Tympanum (tympanic membrane) (see Eardrum)

UCLA Medical Center, 42

University of Iowa Hospitals and Clinics, 42

University of Michigan Medical Center, 42

University of Texas (M. D. Anderson Cancer Center), 42

Vancomycin, 44

Vertigo, 13, 53–55, 69

Very Special Arts, International, 129

Vestibular apparatus, 12

Vestibular Disorders Association of America, 129

Vestibuloocular system, 12

Volume, 9, 26

Vowels, 8, 17, 26

ABOUT THE AUTHOR

Norra Tannenhaus holds degrees in biopsychology and nutrition from Vassar College and Columbia University. She has written extensively on health, medicine, and nutrition for consumers and physicians, and her magazine articles have appeared in such major publications as *Self, Glamour,* and *Mademoiselle. What You Can Do About Hearing Loss* is her eighth book. She is the author of several other titles in the Dell Medical Library, including *Learning to Live with Chronic IBS* and *What You Can Do About Diabetes.*